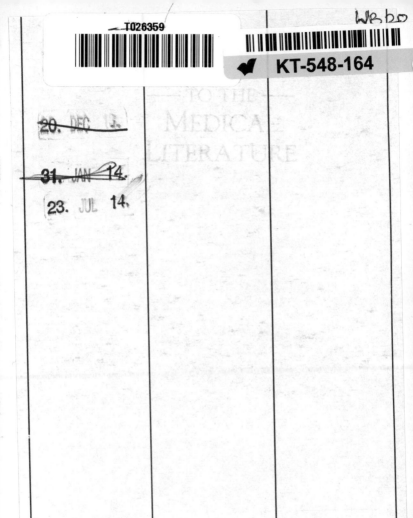

Notice

Medicine is an ever-changing science. As new research and clinical experience broaden our knowledge, changes in treatment and drug therapy are required. The authors and the publisher of this work have checked with sources believed to be reliable in their efforts to provide information that is complete and generally in accord with the standards accepted at the time of publication. However, in view of the possibility of human error or changes in medical sciences, neither the authors nor the publisher nor any other party who has been involved in the preparation or publication of this work warrants that the information contained herein is in every respect accurate or complete, and they disclaim all responsibility for any errors or omissions or for the results obtained from use of the information contained in this work. Readers are encouraged to confirm the information contained herein with other sources. For example and in particular, readers are advised to check the product information sheet included in the package of each drug they plan to administer to be certain that the information contained in this work is accurate and that changes have not been made in the recommended dose or in the contraindications for administration. This recommendation is of particular importance in connection with new or infrequently used drugs.

USERS' GUIDES
—— TO THE ——
MEDICAL
LITERATURE

ESSENTIALS OF EVIDENCE-BASED CLINICAL PRACTICE
SECOND EDITION

The Evidence-Based Medicine Working Group
Editors

Gordon Guyatt, MD, MSc
Departments of Clinical
   Epidemiology and Biostatistics
   and Medicine
Faculty of Health Sciences
McMaster University
Hamilton, Ontario, Canada

**Maureen O. Meade, MD,
FRCPC, MSc**
Departments of Medicine and
   Clinical Epidemiology and
   Biostatistics
Faculty of Health Sciences
McMaster University
Hamilton, Ontario, Canada

Drummond Rennie, MD
JAMA
Chicago, Illinois
Philip R. Lee Institute for Health
   Policy Studies
University of California,
   San Francisco
San Francisco, California, USA

Deborah J. Cook, MD, MSc
Departments of Medicine and
   Clinical Epidemiology and
   Biostatistics
Faculty of Health Sciences
McMaster University
Hamilton, Ontario, Canada

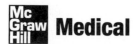

New York Chicago San Francisco Lisbon
London Madrid Mexico City Milan New Delhi
San Juan Seoul Singapore Sydney Toronto

JAMAevidence

JAMA
& ARCHIVES
JOURNALS
American Medical Association

The McGraw·Hill Companies

7 8 9 0 DOC/DOC 14 13

Set: ISBN 978-0-07-159038-9; MHID 0-07-159038-2
Book: ISBN 978-0-07-159040-2; MHID 0-07-159040-4
Pocket Cards: ISBN 978-0-07-160850-3; MHID 0-07-160850-8

JAMA and *Archives* Journals:
Editor in Chief: Catherine D. DeAngelis, MD, MPH
Executive Deputy Editor: Phil B. Fontanarosa, MD, MBA
Managing Deputy Editor: Annette Flanagin, RN, MA
Manuscript Editor: Cara Wallace

McGraw-Hill Professional:
This book was set in Minion and Zurich by Silverchair Science + Communications, Inc.
The editors were James F. Shanahan and Robert Pancotti.
The production supervisor was Philip Galea.
The illustration manager was Armen Ovsepyan.
Project management was provided by Pete Compitello, The Egerton Group, Ltd.
The cover designer was The Gazillion Group.
Cover photograph by Brand X Photography.
RR Donnelley was printer and binder.
This book is printed on acid-free paper.

Library of Congress Cataloging-in-Publication Data

Users' guides to the medical literature : essentials of evidence-based clinical practice / edited
by Gordon Guyatt, Drummond Rennie, Maureen O. Meade, Deborah J. Cook—2nd ed.
    p. ; cm.
  Rev. ed. of: Users' guides to the medical literature : essentials of evidence-based clinical
practice / edited by Gordon Guyatt, Drummond Rennie. c2002.
  Includes bibliographical references and index.
  ISBN-13: 978-0-07-159038-9 (pbk. : alk. paper)
  ISBN-10: 0-07-159038-2 (pbk. : alk. paper)
  1. Evidence-based medicine. 2. Clinical medicine. I. Guyatt, Gordon. II. Rennie, Drummond.
III. Meade, Maureen O. IV. Cook, Deborah J. V. Title: Essentials of evidence-based clinical
practice.
  [DNLM: 1. Evidence-Based Medicine. 2. Clinical Medicine. 3. Decision Making.
4. Diagnosis, Differential. 5. Review Literature as Topic. WB 102 U84 2008]
RA427.U84 2008
616—dc22   2007047779

To our students, in many countries, whose interest, passion, and probing questions made possible the development of the methods we use to communicate the concepts of evidence-based medicine.

GG, MOM, and DJC

To Deb, who has watched over and tended me while I have watched over and tended this wonderful group of authors, with gratitude for her love and her good humor.

DR

CONTENTS

JAMAevidence: Using Evidence to Improve Care

Founded around the *Users' Guides to the Medical Literature* and *The Rational Clinical Examination: Evidence-Based Clinical Diagnosis*, JAMAevidence offers an invaluable online resource for learning, teaching, and practicing evidence-based medicine. Updated regularly, the site includes fully searchable content of the *Users' Guides to the Medical Literature* and *The Rational Clinical Examination* and features podcasts from the leading minds in EBM, interactive worksheets, question wizards, functional calculators, and a comprehensive collection of PowerPoint slides for educators and students.

www.JAMAevidence.com

Please visit the following Web site for information on subscription rates: www.mhprofessional.com/jama

JAMA
&
ARCHIVES
JOURNALS
American Medical Association

Contributors

Alexandra Barratt, MBBS, FAFPHM, MPH, PhD
Department of Epidemiology
School of Public Health
University of Sydney
Sydney, New South Wales,
    Australia

Heiner C. Bucher, MD
Clinical Epidemiology
Basel Institute for Clinical
    Epidemiology
University Hospital Basel
Basel, Switzerland

Deborah J. Cook, MD, MSc
Departments of Medicine and
    Clinical Epidemiology and
    Biostatistics
Faculty of Health Sciences
McMaster University
Hamilton, Ontario, Canada

P. J. Devereaux, BSc, MD, PhD
Departments of Clinical
    Epidemiology and
    Biostatistics and Medicine
McMaster University
Hamilton, Ontario, Canada

Toshi A. Furukawa, MD, PhD
Department of Psychiatry and
    Cognitive-Behavioral
    Medicine
Nagoya City University Graduate
    School of Medical Sciences
Nagoya, Japan

Gordon Guyatt, MD, MSc
Chair, Evidence-Based Medicine
    Working Group
Departments of Clinical
    Epidemiology and
    Biostatistics and Medicine
Faculty of Health Sciences
McMaster University
Hamilton, Ontario, Canada

Ted Haines, MD, MSc
Departments of Clinical
    Epidemiology and Biostatistics
    and Occupational Health
    Program
McMaster University
Hamilton, Ontario, Canada

Brian Haynes, MD, MSc, PhD
Department of Clinical
    Epidemiology and
    Biostatistics
McMaster University
Hamilton, Ontario, Canada

Dereck Hunt, MD, MSc, FRCPC
Health Information Research Unit
Henderson General Hospital
Hamilton, Ontario, Canada

John P. A. Ioannidis, MD, PhD
Department of Hygiene and
    Epidemiology
University of Ioannina School of
    Medicine
Ioannina, Greece
Department of Medicine
Tufts University School of
    Medicine
Boston, Massachusetts, USA

Roman Jaeschke, MD, MSc
Department of Medicine
McMaster University
Hamilton, Ontario, Canada

Regina Kunz, MD, PhD
Basel Institute for Clinical
    Epidemiology
University Hospital Basel
Basel, Switzerland

Mitchell Levine, MD, MSc
Centre for Evaluation of Medicines
St. Joseph's Healthcare
Hamilton, Ontario, Canada

Thomas G. McGinn, MD, MPH
Department of General Internal
    Medicine
Mount Sinai School of Medicine
New York, New York, USA

Ann McKibbon, MLS, PhD
Department of Clinical
    Epidemiology and Biostatistics
Health Information Research Unit
McMaster University
Hamilton, Ontario, Canada

Maureen O. Meade, MD, FRCPC, MSc
Departments of Medicine and
    Clinical Epidemiology and
    Biostatistics
Faculty of Health Sciences
McMaster University
Hamilton, Ontario, Canada

Victor Montori, MD
Department of Medicine
Knowledge and Encounter
    Research Unit
Mayo Clinic and Foundation
Rochester, Minnesota, USA

Kameshwar Prasad, MD, DM, MMSc
Clinical Epidemiology Unit
All India Institute of Medical
    Sciences
New Delhi, India

Adrienne Randolph, MD, MSc
Department of Anesthesia,
    Perioperative and Pain
    Medicine
Children's Hospital Boston
Harvard Medical School
Boston, Massachusetts, USA

Drummond Rennie, MD
JAMA
Chicago, Illinois
Philip R. Lee Institute for Health
  Policy Studies
University of California, San
  Francisco
San Francisco, California, USA

Scott Richardson, MD
Department of Internal
  Medicine
Wright State University
Dayton, Ohio, USA

Holger J. Schünemann, MD
Department of Epidemiology
Italian National Cancer Institute
  Regina Elena
Rome, Italy
Departments of Medicine and
  Social and Preventive Medicine
State University of New York at
  Buffalo
Buffalo, New York, USA

Sharon Straus, MD
Department of Medicine
University of Calgary
Calgary, Alberta, Canada
University of Toronto
Toronto, Ontario, Canada

Stephen Walter, PhD
Department of Clinical
  Epidemiology and Biostatistics
McMaster University
Hamilton, Ontario, Canada

Mark C. Wilson, MD, MPH
Department of Internal
  Medicine
University of Iowa Hospitals and
  Clinics
Iowa City, Iowa, USA

Peter Wyer, MD
Department of Medicine
Columbia University College of
  Physicians and Surgeons
New York, New York, USA

FOREWORD

When I was attending school in wartime Britain, staples of the curriculum, along with cold baths, mathematics, boiled cabbage, and long cross-country runs, were Latin and French. It was obvious that Latin was a theoretical exercise—the Romans were dead, after all. However, although France was clearly visible just across the Channel, for years it was either occupied or inaccessible, so learning the French language seemed just as impractical and theoretical an exercise. It was unthinkable to me and my teachers that I would ever put it to practical use—that French was a language to be spoken.

This is the relationship too many practitioners have with the medical literature—clearly visible but utterly inaccessible. We recognize that practice should be based on discoveries announced in the medical journals. But we also recognize that every few years the literature doubles in size, and every year we seem to have less time to weigh it,[1] so every day the task of taming the literature becomes more hopeless. The translation of those hundreds of thousands of articles into everyday practice appears to be an obscure task left to others. And as the literature becomes more inaccessible, so does the idea that the literature has any utility for a particular patient become more fanciful.

This book, now in its second edition, is designed to change all that. It's designed to make the clinician fluent in the language of the medical literature in all its forms. To free the clinician from practicing medicine by rote, by guesswork, and by their variably-integrated experience. To put a stop to clinicians being ambushed by drug company representatives, or by their patients, telling them of new therapies the clinicians are unable to evaluate. To end their dependence on out-of-date authority. To enable the practitioner to work from the patient and use the literature as a tool to solve the patient's problems. To provide the clinician access to what is relevant and the ability to assess its validity and whether it applies to a specific patient. In other words, to put the clinician in charge of the single most powerful resource in medicine.

The Users' Guides Series in *JAMA*

I have left it to Gordon Guyatt, MD, MSc, the moving force, principal editor, and most prolific coauthor of the "Users' Guides to the Medical Literature" series in *JAMA*, to describe the history of this series and of this book in the accompanying preface. But where did *JAMA* come into this story?

In the late 1980s, at the invitation of my friend David Sackett, MD, I visited his department at McMaster University to discuss a venture with *JAMA*—a series examining the evidence behind the clinical history and examination. After these discussions, a series of articles and systematic reviews was developed and, with the enthusiastic support of then *JAMA* editor in chief George Lundberg, MD, *JAMA* began publishing the Rational Clinical Examination series in 1992.[2] By that time, I had formed an excellent working relationship with the brilliant group at McMaster. Like their leader, Sackett, they tended to be iconoclastic, expert at working together and forming alliances with new and talented workers, and intellectually exacting. Like their leader, they delivered on their promises.

So, when I heard that they were thinking of updating the wonderful little series of Readers' Guides published in 1981 in the *Canadian Medical Association Journal*, I took advantage of this working relationship to urge them to update and expand the series for *JAMA*. Together with Sackett, and first with Andy Oxman, MD, and then with Gordon Guyatt taking the lead (when Oxman left to take a position in Oslo), the Users' Guides to the Medical Literature series was born. We began publishing articles in the series in *JAMA* in 1993.[3]

At the start, we thought we might have 8 or 10 articles, but the response from readers was so enthusiastic, and the variety of types of article in the literature so great, that 7 years later I still found myself receiving, sending for review, and editing new articles for the series. Just before the first edition of this book was published, Gordon Guyatt and I closed this series at 25, appearing as 33 separate journal articles.

The passage of years during the preparation of the original *JAMA* series and the publication of the first edition of this book had a particularly useful result. Some subjects that were scarcely discussed in the major medical journals in the early 1990s, but that had burgeoned years later, could receive the attention that had become their due. For instance, in 2000, *JAMA* published 2 users' guides[4,5] on how readers should approach reports of qualitative research in health care. To take another example, systematic reviews and meta-analyses, given a huge boost by the activities of the Cochrane Collaboration, had become prominent features of the literature. An article in the series,[6] first published in 1994, discusses how to use such studies. Another example would be the guide on electronic health information resources,[7] first published in 2000. Each of these users' guides has been reviewed and thoroughly updated for this second edition.

The Book

From the start, readers kept urging us to put the series together as a book. That had been our intention right from the start, but each new article delayed its implementation. How fortunate! When the original Readers' Guides appeared in the *CMAJ* in 1981, Gordon Guyatt's phrase "evidence-based medicine" had never been coined, and only a tiny proportion of health care workers possessed computers. The Internet did not exist and electronic publication was only a dream. In 1992, the Web—for practical purposes—had scarcely been invented, the dot-com bubble had not appeared, let alone burst, and the health professions were only beginning to become computer literate. But at the end of the 1990s, when Guyatt and I approached my colleagues at *JAMA* with the idea of publishing not merely the standard printed book but also Web-based and CD-ROM formats of the book, they were immediately receptive. Putting the latter part into practice has been the notable achievement of Rob Hayward, MD, of the Centre for Health Evidence of the University of Alberta.

The science and art of evidence-based medicine, which this book does so much to reinforce, has developed remarkably during the past 2 decades, and this is reflected in every page of this book. Encouraged by the immediate success of the first edition of the *Users' Guides*, Gordon Guyatt and the Evidence-Based Medicine

Working Group have once again brought each chapter up to date for this second edition.

An updated Web version of the *Users' Guides to the Medical Literature* will accompany the new edition, building upon the excellent work completed by Rob Hayward and his colleagues at the Centre for Health Evidence, University of Alberta, Edmonton. As part of a new online educational resource entitled JAMAevidence, the second edition of the *Users' Guides* online will be intertwined online with the first edition of the *Rational Clinical Examination: Evidence-Based Clinical Diagnosis*. Together they will serve as the cornerstones of a comprehensive online educational resource for teaching and learning evidence-based medicine. Interactive calculators and worksheets will provide practical complements to the content, while downloadable PowerPoint presentations will serve as invaluable resources for instructors. Finally, podcast presentations will bring the foremost minds behind evidence-based medicine to medical students, residents, and faculty around the world.

Once again, I thank Gordon Guyatt for being an inspired author, a master organizer, and a wonderful teacher, colleague, and friend. I know personally and greatly admire a good number of his colleagues in the Evidence-Based Medicine Working Group, but it would be invidious to name them, given the huge collective effort this has entailed. This is an enterprise that came about only because of the strenuous efforts of many individuals. On the *JAMA* side, I must thank Annette Flanagin, RN, MA, a wonderfully efficient, creative, and diplomatic colleague at *JAMA*. I also wish to thank Barry Bowlus, Joanne Spatz, Margaret Winker, MD, and Richard Newman of the *JAMA* and *Archives* Journals, who have made important contributions. In addition, I acknowledge the efforts of our partners at McGraw-Hill Medical—James Shanahan, Robert Pancotti, Scott Grillo, and Helen Parr.

Finally, I thank Cathy DeAngelis, MD, MPH, editor in chief of the *JAMA* and *Archives* Journals, for her strong backing of me, my colleagues, and this project; for her tolerance; and for keeping up everyone's spirits with her dreadful jokes. Throughout, Cathy has guided the project forward with wisdom, humor, and understanding, and we are all grateful.

Drummond Rennie, MD

JAMA

University of California, San Francisco

References

1. Durack DT. The weight of medical knowledge. *N Engl J Med*. 1978;298 (14):773-775.

2. Sackett DL, Rennie D. The science of the art of the clinical examination. *JAMA*. 1992;267(19):2650-2652.

3. Guyatt GH, Rennie D. Users' guides to the medical literature. *JAMA*. 1993;270(17):2096-2097.

4. Giacomini MK, Cook DJ; Evidence-Based Medicine Working Group. Users' guides to the medical literature, XXIII: qualitative research in health care A: are the results of the study valid? *JAMA*. 2000;284(3):357-362.

5. Giacomini MK, Cook DJ; Evidence-Based Medicine Working Group. Users' guides to the medical literature, XXIII: qualitative research in health care B: what are the results and how do they help me care for my patients? *JAMA*. 2000;284(4):478-482.

6. Oxman AD, Cook DJ, Guyatt GH; Evidence-Based Medicine Working Group. Users' guides to the medical literature, VI: how to use an overview. *JAMA*. 1994;272(17):1367-1371.

7. Hunt DL, Jaeschke R, McKibbon KA; Evidence-Based Medicine Working Group. Users' guides to the medical literature, XXI: using electronic health information resources in evidence-based practice. *JAMA*. 2000;283(14): 1875-1879.

PREFACE

In fewer than 20 years, evidence-based medicine (EBM) has gone from a tentative name of a fledgling concept to the fundamental basis for clinical practice that is used worldwide. The first history of the movement has already appeared in the form of an authoritative book.[1] This second edition of *Users' Guides to the Medical Literature* reflects that history and the evolving conceptual and pedagogic basis of the EBM movement.

In 1981, a group of clinical epidemiologists at McMaster University, led by Dave Sackett, published the first of a series of articles advising clinicians how to read clinical journals.[2] Although a huge step forward, the series had its limitations. After teaching what they then called "critical appraisal" for a number of years, the group became increasingly aware of both the necessity and the challenges of going beyond reading the literature in a browsing mode and using research studies to solve patient management problems on a day-to-day basis.

In 1990, I assumed the position of residency director of the Internal Medicine Program at McMaster. Through Dave Sackett's leadership, critical appraisal had evolved into a philosophy of medical practice based on knowledge and understanding of the medical literature (or lack of such knowledge and understanding) supporting each clinical decision. We believed that this represented a fundamentally different style of practice and required a term that would capture this difference.

My mission as residency director was to train physicians who would practice this new approach to medical practice. In the spring of 1990, I presented our plans for changing the program to the members of the Department of Medicine, many of whom were not sympathetic. The term suggested to describe the new approach was *scientific medicine*. Those already hostile were incensed and disturbed at the implication that they had previously been "unscientific." My second try at a name for our philosophy of medical practice, *evidence-based medicine*, turned out to be a catchy one.

EBM first appeared in the autumn of 1990 in an information document for residents entering, or considering application to, the residency program. The relevant passage follows:

> Residents are taught to develop an attitude of "enlightened scepticism" towards the application of diagnostic, therapeutic, and prognostic technologies in their day-to-day management of patients. This approach…has been called "evidence-based medicine".… The goal is to be aware of the evidence on which one's practice is based, the soundness of the evidence, and the strength of inference the evidence permits. The strategy employed requires a clear delineation of the relevant question(s); a thorough search of the literature relating to the questions; a critical appraisal of the evidence and its applicability to the clinical situation; a balanced application of the conclusions to the clinical problem.

The first published appearance of the term was in the American College of Physicians' Journal Club in 1991.[3] Meanwhile, our group of enthusiastic evidence-based medical educators at McMaster, including Brian Haynes, Deborah J. Cook, and Roman Jaeschke, were refining our practice and teaching of EBM. Believing that we were on to something big, the McMaster folks linked up with a larger group of academic physicians, largely from the United States, to form the first Evidence-Based Medicine Working Group and published an article that expanded greatly on the description of EBM, labeling it as a "paradigm shift."[4]

This working group then addressed the task of producing a new set of articles, the successor to the readers' guides, to present a more practical approach to applying the medical literature to clinical practice. Although a large number of people made important contributions, the non-McMaster folks who provided the greatest input to the intensive development of educational strategies included Scott Richardson, Mark Wilson, Rob Hayward, and Virginia Moyer. With the unflagging support and wise counsel of *JAMA* deputy editor Drummond Rennie, the Evidence-Based Medicine Working Group created a 25-part series called the Users' Guides to the Medical Literature, published in *JAMA* between 1993 and 2000.[5] The first edition of the *Users' Guides* was a direct descendant of the *JAMA* series and this second edition represents its latest incarnation.

It didn't take long for people to realize that the principles of EBM were equally applicable for other health care workers including nurses, dentists, orthodontists, physiotherapists, occupational therapists, chiropractors, and podiatrists. Thus, terms such as *evidence-based health care* or *evidence-based practice* are appropriate to cover the full range of clinical applications of the evidence-based approach to patient care. Because this book is directed primarily to physicians, we have stayed with the term EBM.

This edition of *Users' Guides to the Medical Literature* presents what we have learned from our students in 25 years of teaching the concepts of EBM. Thanks to the interest, enthusiasm, and diversity of our students, we are able to present the material with increasing clarity and identify more compelling examples. For more than 10 years, our group has hosted a workshop called How to Teach Evidence-Based Practice at McMaster. At the workshop, more than 100 EBM teachers from around the world, at various stages of their careers as educators, engage in a week of mutual education. They share their experiences, communicating EBM concepts to undergraduate and graduate students, residents and fellows, and colleagues. Invariably, even the most senior of us come away with new and better ways of helping students to actively learn EBM's underlying principles.

We are also blessed with the opportunity to travel the world, helping to teach at other people's EBM workshops. Participating in workshops in Thailand, Saudi Arabia, Egypt, Pakistan, Oman, Singapore, the Philippines, Japan, Peru, Chile, Brazil, Germany, Spain, France, Belgium, Norway, and Switzerland—the list goes on—provides us with an opportunity to try out and refine our teaching approaches with students who have a tremendous heterogeneity of backgrounds and perspectives. At each of these workshops, the local EBM teachers share their own experiences, struggles, accomplishments, and EBM teaching tips that we can add to our repertoire.

We are grateful for the extraordinary privilege of sharing, in the form of the second edition of *Users' Guides to the Medical Literature*, what we have learned.

Gordon Guyatt, MD, MSc
McMaster University

References

1. Daly J. *Evidence-Based Medicine and the Search for a Science of Clinical Care*. Berkeley, CA: Milbank Memorial Fund and University of California Press; 2005.

2. How to read clinical journals, I: why to read them and how to start reading them critically. *CMAJ*. 1981;124(5):555-558.

3. Guyatt G. Evidence-based medicine. *ACP J Club (Ann Intern Med)*. 1991; 114(suppl 2):A-16.

4. Evidence-Based Medicine Working Group. Evidence-based medicine: a new approach to teaching the practice of medicine. *JAMA*. 1992;268(17): 2420-2425.

5. Guyatt GH, Rennie D. Users' guides to the medical literature. *JAMA*. 1993;270(17):2096-2097.

HOW TO USE THE MEDICAL LITERATURE— AND THIS BOOK— TO IMPROVE YOUR PATIENT CARE

Gordon Guyatt and Maureen O. Meade

IN THIS CHAPTER:

The Structure of the Users' Guides

The Approach of the *Users' Guides to the Medical Literature*

The objective of this book is to help you make efficient use of the published literature to guide your patient care. What does the published literature comprise? Our definition is broad. You may find *evidence* in a wide variety of sources, including original journal articles, *reviews* and *synopses* of *primary studies*, *practice guidelines*, and traditional and innovative medical textbooks. Increasingly, clinicians can most easily access many of these sources through the World Wide Web. In the future, the Internet may be the only route of access for some resources.

THE STRUCTURE OF THE *USERS' GUIDES*

This book is not like a novel that you read through from beginning to end. Indeed, the *Users' Guides* is designed so that each chapter is largely self-contained. Thus, we anticipate that clinicians may be selective in their reading. You are also likely to find the glossary of terms a useful reminder of formal definition of terms used in the book. All terms in the glossary appear in italics in the text.

THE APPROACH OF THE *USERS' GUIDES TO THE MEDICAL LITERATURE*

The structure of this book reflects how we believe you should go about using the literature to provide optimal patient care. Our approach to addressing diagnosis, treatment, *harm*, and *prognosis* begins when the clinician faces a clinical dilemma (Figure 1-1). Having identified the problem, the clinician then formulates a structured clinical question (see Chapter 3, What Is the Question?) and continues with finding the best relevant evidence (see Chapter 4, Finding the Evidence) (Figure 1-1).

FIGURE 1-1

Approach to Addressing Diagnosis, Treatment, Harm, and Prognosis

Identify your problem.
↓
Define a structured question.
↓
Find the best evidence.
(original primary study or evidence summary)
↓
How valid is the evidence?
↓
What are the results?
↓
How should I apply the results to patient care?

Most chapters of this book include an example search for the best evidence. These searches are accurate at the time they were done, but you are unlikely to get exactly the same results if you replicate the searches now. Reasons include additions to the literature and occasional structural changes in databases. Thus, you should view the searches as illustrations of searching principles, rather than as currently definitive searches addressing the clinical question.

Having identified the best evidence, the clinician then proceeds through 3 steps in evaluating that evidence (Figure 1-1). The first step asks, Are the results of the study *valid*? This question has to do with the believability of the results. Another way to state this question is: Do these results represent an unbiased estimate of the truth, or have they been influenced in some systematic fashion to lead to a false conclusion?

In the second step (What are the results?), we consider the size and precision of the *treatment effect* from randomized trials (therapy) (see Chapter 6, Therapy [Randomized Trials]; Chapter 7, Does Treatment Lower Risk? Understanding the Results; and Chapter 8,

Confidence Intervals), the evidence that helps us generate *pretest probabilities* and move to *posttest probabilities* on the basis of test results (diagnosis) (see Chapter 11, Differential Diagnosis; and Chapter 12, Diagnostic Tests), the size and precision of our estimate of a harmful effect from observational studies (harm) (see Chapter 9, Harm [Observational Studies]), and our best estimate of a patient's fate (prognosis) (see Chapter 13, Prognosis).

Once we understand the results, we can ask ourselves the third question, How can I apply these results to patient care? This question has 2 parts. First, can you *generalize* (or, to put it another way, particularize) the results to your patient? For instance, you should hesitate to institute a treatment if your patient is too dissimilar from those who participated in the trial or trials. Second, if the results are generalizable to your patient, what is the significance for your patient? Have the investigators measured all *outcomes* of importance to patients? The effect of an intervention depends on both benefits and *risks* of alternative management strategies.

To help demonstrate the clinical relevance of this approach, we begin each core chapter with a clinical scenario, demonstrate a search for relevant literature, and present a table that summarizes criteria for assessing the validity, results, and applicability of the article of interest. We then address the clinical scenario applying the validity, results, and applicability criteria to an article from the medical literature.

Experience on the wards and outpatient clinics, and with the first edition of the *Users' Guide*, has taught us that this approach is well suited to the needs of any clinician who is eager to achieve an evidence-based practice.

THE PHILOSOPHY OF EVIDENCE-BASED MEDICINE

Gordon Guyatt, Brian Haynes, Roman Jaeschke,
Maureen O. Meade, Mark Wilson, Victor Montori,
and Scott Richardson

Evidence-based medicine (EBM) is about solving clinical problems. In 1992, we described EBM as a shift in medical paradigms.[1] In contrast to the traditional paradigm of medical practice, EBM places lower value on unsystematic clinical experience and pathophysiologic rationale, stresses the examination of *evidence* from clinical research, suggests that interpreting the results of clinical research requires a formal set of rules, and places a lower value on authority than the traditional medical paradigm. Although we continue to find this paradigm shift a valid way of conceptualizing EBM, the world is often complex enough to invite more than 1 useful way of thinking about an idea or a phenomenon. In this chapter, we describe another conceptualization that emphasizes how EBM complements and enhances the traditional skills of clinical practice.

TWO FUNDAMENTAL PRINCIPLES OF EBM

As a distinctive approach to patient care, EBM involves 2 fundamental principles. First, EBM posits a *hierarchy of evidence* to guide clinical decision making. Second, evidence alone is never sufficient to make a clinical decision. Decision makers must always trade off the benefits and *risks*, inconvenience, and costs associated with alternative management strategies and, in doing so, consider their patients' *values* and *preferences*.[1]

A Hierarchy of Evidence

What is the nature of the *evidence* in EBM? We suggest a broad definition: any empirical observation constitutes potential evidence, whether systematically collected or not. Thus, the unsystematic observations of the individual clinician constitute one source of evidence; physiologic experiments constitute another source. Unsystematic observations can lead to profound insights, and wise clinicians develop a healthy respect for the insights of their senior colleagues in issues of clinical observation, diagnosis, and relations with patients and colleagues.

At the same time, our personal clinical observations are often limited by small sample size and by deficiencies in human processes of making inferences.[3] Predictions about *intervention effects* on patient-important outcomes based on physiologic experiments usually are right but occasionally are disastrously wrong. Numerous factors can lead clinicians astray as they try to interpret the results of conventional open trials of therapy. These include *natural history*, *placebo effects*, patient and health worker expectations, and the patient's desire to please.

Given the limitations of unsystematic clinical observations and physiologic rationale, EBM suggests a number of hierarchies of evidence, one of which relates to issues of *prevention* and treatment (Table 2-1).

Issues of diagnosis or *prognosis* require different hierarchies. For instance, *randomization* is not relevant to sorting out how well a test is able to distinguish individuals with a *target condition* or disease from those who are healthy or have a competing condition or disease. For diagnosis, the top of the hierarchy would include studies that enrolled patients about whom clinicians had diagnostic uncertainty and that undertook a *blind* comparison between the candidate test and a *criterion standard* (see Chapter 12, Diagnostic Tests).

TABLE 2-1

Hierarchy of Strength of Evidence for Prevention and Treatment Decisions

- N-of-1 randomized trial
- Systematic reviews of randomized trials
- Single randomized trial
- Systematic review of observational studies addressing patient-important outcomes
- Single observational study addressing patient-important outcomes
- Physiologic studies (studies of blood pressure, cardiac output, exercise capacity, bone density, and so forth)
- Unsystematic clinical observations

Clinical research goes beyond unsystematic clinical observation in providing strategies that avoid or attenuate spurious results. The same strategies that minimize *bias* in conventional therapeutic trials involving multiple patients can guard against misleading results in studies involving single patients.[4] In the *n-of-1 randomized controlled trial* (*n-of-1 RCT*), a patient and clinician are *blind* to whether that patient is receiving active or placebo medication. The patient makes quantitative ratings of troublesome symptoms during each period, and the n-of-1 RCT continues until both the patient and the clinician conclude that the patient is or is not obtaining benefit from the target intervention. N-of-1 RCTs can provide definitive evidence of treatment effectiveness in individual patients[5,6] and may lead to long-term differences in treatment administration.[7] Unfortunately, n-of-1 RCTs are restricted to chronic conditions with treatments that act and cease acting quickly and are subject to considerable logistic challenges. We must therefore usually rely on studies of other patients to make inferences regarding the patient before us.

The requirement that clinicians generalize from results in other people to their patients inevitably weakens inferences about treatment impact and introduces complex issues of how trial results apply to individual patients. Inferences may nevertheless be strong if results come from a *systematic review* of methodologically strong RCTs with consistent results. Inferences generally will be somewhat weaker if only a single RCT is being considered, unless it is large and has enrolled patients much like the patient under consideration (Table 2-1). Because *observational studies* may underestimate or, more typically, overestimate *treatment effects* in an unpredictable fashion,[8,9] their results are far less trustworthy than those of RCTs. Physiologic studies and unsystematic clinical observations provide the weakest inferences about treatment effects.

This hierarchy is not absolute. If treatment effects are sufficiently large and consistent, carefully conducted observational studies may provide more compelling evidence than poorly conducted RCTs. For example, observational studies have allowed extremely strong inferences about the efficacy of penicillin in pneumococcal pneumonia or that of hip replacement in patients with debilitating hip osteoarthritis. Defining the extent to which clinicians should temper the strength of their inferences when only observational studies are available remains one of the important challenges in EBM.

The hierarchy implies a clear course of action for physicians addressing patient problems. They should look for the highest quality available evidence from the hierarchy. The hierarchy makes it clear that any claim that there is no evidence for the effect of a particular treatment is a non sequitur. The evidence may be extremely weak—it may be the unsystematic observation of a single clinician or physiologic studies that point to mechanisms of action that are only indirectly related—but there is always evidence.

Clinical Decision Making: Evidence Is Never Enough

Picture a woman with chronic pain resulting from terminal cancer. She has come to terms with her condition, resolved her affairs, and said her good-byes, and she wishes to receive only palliative care. She develops severe pneumococcal pneumonia. Evidence that antibiotic therapy reduces morbidity and mortality from pneumo-coccal pneumonia is strong. Even evidence this convincing does not, however, dictate that this particular patient should receive antibiotics. Her *values* are such that she would prefer to forgo treatment.

Now picture a second patient, an 85-year-old man with severe dementia who is mute and incontinent, is without family or friends, and spends his days in apparent discomfort. This man develops pneumococcal pneumonia. Although many clinicians would argue that those responsible for his care should not administer antibiotic therapy, others would suggest that they should. Again, evidence of treatment effectiveness does not automatically imply that treatment should be administered.

Finally, picture a third patient, a healthy 30-year-old mother of 2 children who develops pneumococcal pneumonia. No clinician would doubt the wisdom of administering antibiotic therapy to this patient. This does not mean, however, that an underlying value judgment has been unnecessary. Rather, our values are sufficiently concordant, and the benefits so overwhelm the risk of treatment, that the underlying value judgment is unapparent.

By *values* and *preferences*, we mean the collection of goals, expectations, predispositions, and beliefs that individuals have for certain decisions and their potential outcomes. The explicit enumeration and balancing of benefits and risks that are central to EBM brings the underlying value judgments involved in making management decisions into bold relief.

Acknowledging that values play a role in every important patient care decision highlights our limited understanding of how to ensure that decisions are consistent with individual and, where appropriate, societal values. Health economists have played a major role in developing the science of measuring patient preferences.[10,11] Some decision aids incorporate patient values indirectly. If patients truly understand the potential risks and benefits, their decisions will reflect their preferences.[12] These developments constitute a promising start. Nevertheless, many unanswered questions remain concerning how to elicit preferences and how to incorporate them in clinical encounters already subject to crushing time pressures.

Next, we briefly comment on additional skills that clinicians must master for optimal patient care and the relation of those skills to EBM.

CLINICAL SKILLS, HUMANISM, AND EBM

In summarizing the skills and attributes necessary for evidence-based practice, Table 2-2 highlights how EBM complements traditional aspects of clinical expertise. One of us, a secondary-care internist, developed a lesion on his lip shortly before an important presentation. He was concerned and, wondering whether he should take acyclovir, proceeded to spend the next 30 minutes searching for and evaluating the highest-quality evidence. When he began to discuss his remaining uncertainty with his partner, an experienced dentist, she cut short the discussion by exclaiming, "But, my dear, that isn't herpes!"

TABLE 2-2

Knowledge and Skills Necessary for Optimal Evidence-Based Practice

- Diagnostic expertise
- In-depth background knowledge
- Effective searching skills
- Effective critical appraisal skills
- Ability to define and understand benefits and risks of alternatives
- In-depth physiologic understanding allowing application of evidence to the individual
- Sensitivity and communication skills required for full understanding of patient context
- Ability to elicit and understand patient values and preferences and apply them to management decisions

---

This story illustrates the necessity of obtaining the correct diagnosis before seeking and applying research evidence regarding optimal treatment. After making the diagnosis, the clinician relies on experience and background knowledge to define the relevant management options. Having identified those options, the clinician can search for, evaluate, and apply the best evidence regarding treatment.

In applying evidence, clinicians rely on their expertise to define features that affect the applicability of the results to the individual patient. The clinician must judge the extent to which differences in treatment (for instance, local surgical expertise or the possibility of patient *nonadherence*), the availability of monitoring, or patient characteristics (such as age, comorbidity, or the patient's personal circumstances) may affect estimates of benefit and *risk* that come from the published literature.

Understanding the patient's personal circumstances is of particular importance[12] and requires compassion, sensitive listening skills, and broad perspectives from the humanities and social sciences. For some patients, incorporation of patient values for major decisions will mean a full enumeration of the possible benefits, risk, and inconvenience associated with alternative management strategies that are relevant to the particular patient. For some patients and problems, this discussion should involve the patient's family. For other problems—the discussion of *screening* with prostate-specific antigen with older male patients, for instance—attempts to involve other family members might violate strong cultural norms.

Some patients are uncomfortable with an explicit discussion of benefits and risk and object to clinicians placing what they perceive as excessive responsibility for decision making on their shoulders.[13] In such cases, it is the physician's responsibility to develop insight to ensure that choices will be consistent with the patient's values and preferences. Understanding and implementing the sort of decision-making process that patients desire and effectively communicating the information they need require skills in understanding the patient's narrative and the person behind that narrative.[14,15]

ADDITIONAL CHALLENGES FOR EBM

Clinicians will find that time limitations present the biggest challenge to evidence-based practice. Fortunately, new resources to assist clinicians are available and the pace of innovation is rapid. One can consider a classification of information sources that comes with a mnemonic device, 4S: the individual study, the *systematic review* of all the available studies on a given problem, a *synopsis* of both individual studies and summaries, and *systems* of information.[16] By *systems*, we mean summaries that link a number of synopses related to the care of a particular patient problem (acute upper gastrointestinal bleeding) or type of patient (the diabetic outpatient) (Table 2-3). Evidence-based selection and summarization is becoming increasingly available at each level (see Chapter 4, Finding the Evidence).

A second enormous challenge for evidence-based practice is ensuring that management strategies are consistent with the patient's values and preferences. In a time-constrained environment, how can we ensure that patients' involvement in decision

TABLE 2-3

A Hierarchy of Preprocessed Evidence[16]

Studies	Preprocessing involves selecting only those studies that are both highly relevant and characterized by study designs that minimize bias and thus permit a high strength of inference
Systematic reviews	Reviews involving the identification, selection, appraisal, and summary of primary studies addressing a focused clinical question using methods to reduce the likelihood of bias
Synopses	Brief summaries that encapsulate the key methodologic details and results of a single study or systematic review
Systems	Practice guidelines, clinical pathways, or evidence-based textbook summaries that integrate evidence-based information about specific clinical problems and provide regular updates to guide the care of individual patients

making has the form and extent that they desire and that the outcome reflects their needs and desires? Progress in addressing this daunting question will require a major expenditure of time and intellectual energy from clinician researchers.

This book deals primarily with decision making at the level of the individual patient. Evidence-based approaches can also inform health policy making,[17] day-to-day decisions in public health, and systems-level decisions such as those facing hospital managers. In each of these areas, EBM can support the appropriate goal of gaining the greatest health benefit from limited resources.

In the policy arena, dealing with differing values poses even more challenges than in the arena of individual patient care. Should we restrict ourselves to alternative resource allocation within a fixed pool of health care resources, or should we be trading off health care services against, for instance, lower tax rates for individuals or corporations? How should we deal with the large body of observational studies suggesting that social and economic factors may have a larger influence on the health of populations than health care delivery? How should we deal with the tension between what may be best for a person and what may be optimal for the society of which that person is a member? The debate about such issues is at the heart of evidence-based health policy making, but, inevitably, it has implications for decision making at the individual patient level.

References

1. Evidence-Based Medicine Working Group. Evidence-based medicine: a new approach to the teaching of medicine. *JAMA*. 1992;268(17):2420-2425.

2. Napodano R. *Values in Medical Practice.* New York, NY: Humana Sciences Press; 1986.

3. Nisbett R, Ross L. *Human Inference.* Englewood Cliffs, NJ: Prentice-Hall; 1980.

4. Guyatt G, Sackett D, Taylor D, Chong J, Roberts R, Pugsley S. Determining optimal therapy—randomized trials in individual patients. *N Engl J Med.* 1986;314(14):889-892.

5. Guyatt G, Keller J, Jaeschke R, Rosenbloom D, Adachi J, Newhouse M. The n-of-1 randomized controlled trial: clinical usefulness: our three-year experience. *Ann Intern Med.* 1990;112(4):293-299.

6. Larson E, Ellsworth A, Oas J. Randomized clinical trials in single patients during a 2-year period. *JAMA.* 1993;270(22):2708-2712.

7. Mahon J, Laupacis A, Donner A, Wood T. Randomised study of n of 1 trials versus standard practice. *BMJ.* 1996;312(7038):1069-1074.

8. Guyatt G, DiCenso A, Farewell V, Willan A, Griffith L. Randomized trials versus observational studies in adolescent pregnancy prevention. *J Clin Epidemiol.* 2000;53(2):167-174.

9. Kunz R, Oxman A. The unpredictability paradox: review of empirical comparisons of randomised and non-randomised clinical trials. *BMJ.* 1998;317(7167):1185-1190.

10. Drummond M, Richardson W, O'Brien B, Levine M, Heyland D. Users' Guide to the Medical Literature XIII: how to use an article on economic analysis of clinical practice, A: are the results of the study valid? *JAMA.* 1997;277(19):1552-1557.

11. Feeny D, Furlong W, Boyle M, Torrance G. Multi-attribute health status classification systems: health utilities index. *Pharmacoeconomics.* 1995;7(6):490-502.

12. O'Connor A, Rostom A, Fiset V, et al. Decision aids for patients facing health treatment or screening decisions: systematic review. *BMJ.* 1999;319(7212):731-734.

13. Sutherland H, Llewellyn-Thomas H, Lockwood G, Tritchler D, Till J. Cancer patients: their desire for information and participation in treatment decisions. *J R Soc Med.* 1989;82(5):260-263.

14. Greenhalgh T. Narrative based medicine: narrative based medicine in an evidence based world. *BMJ.* 1999;318(7179):323-325.

15. Greenhalgh T, Hurwitz B. Narrative based medicine: why study narrative? *BMJ.* 1999;318(7175):48-50.

16. Haynes R. Of studies, syntheses, synopses, and systems: the "4S" evolution of services for finding current best evidence. *ACP J Club.* 2001;134(2):A11-A13.

17. Muir Gray F, Haynes R, Sackett D, Cook D, Guyatt G. Transferring evidence from research into practice, III: developing evidence-based clinical policy. *ACP J Club.* 1997;126(2):A14-A16.

WHAT IS THE QUESTION?

Gordon Guyatt, Maureen O. Meade,
Scott Richardson, and Roman Jaeschke

IN THIS CHAPTER:

THREE WAYS TO USE THE MEDICAL LITERATURE

Consider a medical student, early in her training, seeing a patient with newly diagnosed diabetes mellitus. She will ask questions such as the following: What is type 2 diabetes mellitus? Why does this patient have polyuria? Why does this patient have numbness and pain in his legs? What treatment options are available? These questions address normal human physiology and the pathophysiology associated with a medical condition.

Traditional medical textbooks that describe underlying physiology, pathology, epidemiology, and general treatment approaches provide an excellent resource for addressing these *background questions*. The sorts of questions that seasoned clinicians usually ask require different resources.

Browsing

A general internist scanning the September/October 2005 *ACP Journal Club* (http://www.acponline.org/journals/acpjc/jcmenu.htm) comes across the following articles: "Intensive Insulin-Glucose Infusion Regimens With Long-Term or Standard Glucose Control Did Not Differ for Reducing Mortality in Type 2 Diabetes Mellitus and MI,"[1] and "Review: Mixed Signals From Trials Concerning Pharmacologic Prevention of Type 2 Diabetes Mellitus."[2]

This internist is in the process of asking a general question—what important new information should I know to optimally treat my patients? Traditionally, clinicians address this question by subscribing to a number of target medical journals in which articles relevant to their practice appear. They keep up to date by skimming the table of contents and reading relevant articles. This traditional approach to what we might call the browsing mode of using the medical literature has major limitations of inefficiency and resulting frustration. *Evidence-based medicine* offers solutions to this problem.

The most efficient strategy is to restrict your browsing to *secondary journals*. For internal and general medicine, *ACP Journal Club* publishes *synopses* of articles that meet criteria of both clinical relevance and methodologic quality. We describe such secondary journals in more detail in Chapter 4, Finding the Evidence.

Some specialties (primary care, mental health) and subspecialties (cardiology, gastroenterology) already have their own devoted secondary journals; others do not. The New York Academy of Medicine keeps a current list of available secondary journals in many health care disciplines (http://www.ebmny.org/journal.html). If you are not yet fortunate enough to have your own, you can apply your own relevance and methodologic screen to articles in your target specialty or subspecialty journals. When you have learned the skills, you will be surprised at the small proportion of studies to which you need attend and at the efficiency with which you can identify them.

Problem Solving

Experienced clinicians confronting a patient with diabetes mellitus will ask questions such as, In patients with new-onset type 2 diabetes mellitus, which clinical features or test results predict the development of diabetic complications? In patients with type 2 diabetes mellitus requiring drug therapy, does starting with metformin treatment yield improved diabetes control and reduce long-term complications better than other initial treatments? Here, clinicians are defining specific questions raised in caring for patients and then consulting the literature to resolve these questions.

Background and Foreground Questions

One can think of the first set of questions, those of the medical student, as *background questions* and of the browsing and problem-solving sets as *foreground questions*. In most situations, you need to understand the background thoroughly before it makes sense to address foreground issues.

A seasoned clinician may occasionally require background information, which is most likely when a new condition or medical *syndrome* appears ("What is SARS?") or when a new diagnostic test ("How does PCR work?") or treatment modality ("What are atypical antipsychotic agents?") appears in the clinical arena.

FIGURE 3-1

Background and Foreground Questions

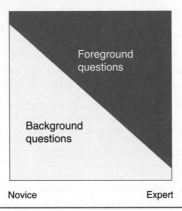

Foreground
questions

Background
questions

Novice   Expert

Figure 3-1 represents the evolution of the questions we ask as we progress from being novices posing background questions to experts posing foreground questions. This book explores how clinicians can use the medical literature to solve their foreground questions.

CLARIFYING YOUR QUESTION

The Structure: Patients, Exposure, Outcome
Clinical questions often spring to mind in a form that makes finding answers in the medical literature a challenge. Dissecting the question into its component parts to facilitate finding the best *evidence* is a fundamental skill.[2] One can divide most questions into 3 parts: the patients, the intervention or *exposure*, and the *outcome* (Table 3-1).

Five Types of Clinical Questions
In addition to clarifying the population, intervention or exposures, and outcome, it is productive to label the nature of the question

TABLE 3-1

Framing Clinical Questions

1. *The population*. Who are the relevant patients?

2. *The interventions or exposures* (diagnostic tests, foods, drugs, surgical procedures, time, risk factors, etc). What are the management strategies we are interested in comparing or the potentially harmful exposures about which we are concerned? For issues of therapy, prevention, or harm, there will always be both an experimental intervention or putative harmful exposure and a control, alternative, or comparison intervention or state to which it is compared.

3. *The outcome*. What are the patient-relevant consequences of the exposures in which we are interested? We may also be interested in the consequences to society, including cost or resource use. It may also be important to specify the period of interest.

that you are asking. There are 5 fundamental types of clinical questions:

1. Therapy: determining the effect of interventions on *patient-important outcomes* (*symptoms*, function, morbidity, mortality, costs)

2. Harm: ascertaining the effects of potentially harmful agents (including therapies from the first type of question) on patient-important outcomes

3. Differential diagnosis: in patients with a particular clinical presentation, establishing the frequency of the underlying disorders

4. Diagnosis: establishing the *power* of a test to differentiate between those with and without a *target condition* or disease

5. Prognosis: estimating a patient's future course

Finding a Suitably Designed Study for Your Question Type

You need to correctly identify the category of study because, to answer your question, you must find an appropriately designed study. If you look for a *randomized trial* to inform you of the properties of a diagnostic test, you are unlikely to find the answer you seek. We will now review the study designs associated with the 5 major types of questions.

To answer questions about a therapeutic issue, we identify studies in which a process analogous to flipping a coin determines participants' receipt of an *experimental treatment* or a control or standard treatment, a *randomized controlled trial* (*RCT*) (see Chapter 6, Therapy [Randomized Trials]). Once investigators allocate participants to treatment or *control groups*, they follow them forward in time to determine whether they have, for instance, a stroke or heart attack—what we call the outcome of interest (Figure 3-2).

Ideally, we would also look to randomized trials to address issues of *harm*. For many potentially harmful exposures, however, randomly allocating patients is neither practical nor ethical. For instance, one cannot suggest to potential study participants that an investigator will decide by the flip of a coin whether or not they smoke during the next 20 years. For exposures like smoking, the best one can do is identify studies in which personal choice, or happenstance, determines whether people are exposed or not exposed. These *observational studies* (often subclassified as *cohort* or *case-control studies*) provide weaker evidence than randomized trials (see Chapter 9, Harm [Observational Studies]).

FIGURE 3-2

Structure of Randomized Trials

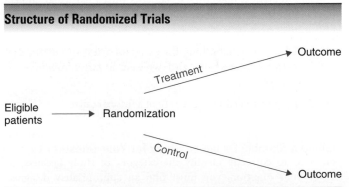

FIGURE 3-3

Structure of Observational Cohort Studies

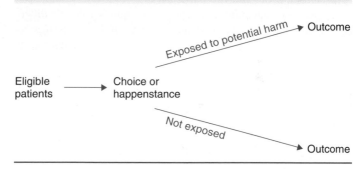

Figure 3-3 depicts a common observational study design in which patients with and without the exposures of interest are followed forward in time to determine whether they experience the outcome of interest. For smoking, one important outcome would likely be the development of cancer.

For sorting out *differential diagnosis*, we need a different study design (Figure 3-4). Here, investigators collect a group of patients with a similar presentation (painless jaundice, syncope, headache), conduct an extensive battery of tests, and, if necessary, follow patients forward in time. Ultimately, for each patient they hope to

FIGURE 3-4

Structure for Studies of Differential Diagnosis

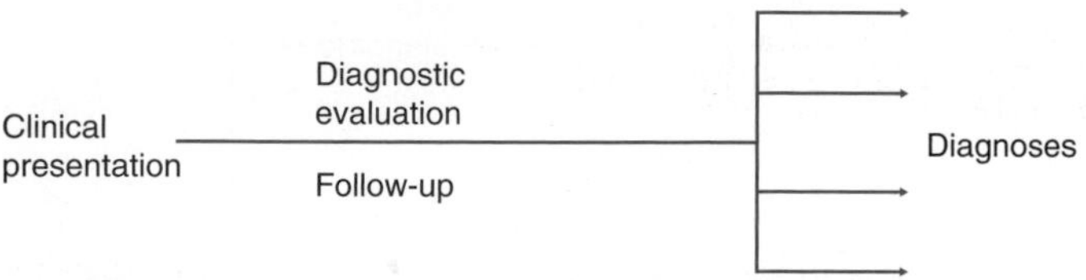

establish the underlying cause of the *symptoms* and *signs* with which the patient presented.

Establishing the value of a particular diagnostic test (what we call its properties or operating characteristics) requires a slightly different design (Figure 3-5). In diagnostic test studies, investigators identify a group of patients in whom they suspect a disease or condition of interest exists (such as tuberculosis, lung cancer, or iron-deficiency anemia), which we call the target condition. These patients undergo the new diagnostic test and a *reference standard*, *gold standard*, or *criterion standard*. Investigators evaluate the diagnostic test by comparing its classification of patients with that of the reference standard (Figure 3-5).

A final type of study examines a patient's *prognosis* and may identify factors that modify that prognosis. Here, investigators identify patients who belong to a particular group (such as pregnant women, patients undergoing surgery, or patients with cancer) with or without factors that may modify their prognosis (such as age or *comorbidity*). The exposure here is time, and investigators follow patients to determine whether they experience the *target outcome*, such as a problem birth at the end of a pregnancy, a myocardial infarction after surgery, or survival in cancer (Figure 3-6).

FIGURE 3-5

Structure for Studies of Diagnostic Test Properties

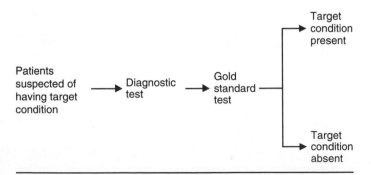

FIGURE 3-6

Structure of Studies of Prognosis

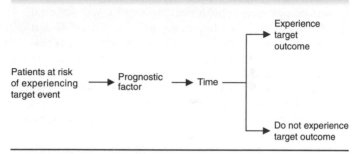

Three Examples of Question Clarification

We will now provide examples of the transformation of unstructured clinical questions into the structured questions that facilitate the use of the medical literature.

Example 1: Diabetes and Target Blood Pressure

A 55-year-old white woman presents with type 2 diabetes mellitus and hypertension. Her glycemic control is excellent with metformin, and she has no history of complications. To manage her hypertension, she takes a small daily dose of a thiazide diuretic. During a 6-month period, her blood pressure is near 155/88 mm Hg.

Initial Question: When treating hypertension, at what target blood pressure should we aim?

Digging Deeper: One limitation of this formulation of the question is that it fails to specify the population in adequate detail. The benefits of tight control of blood pressure may differ in diabetic patients vs nondiabetic patients, in type 1 vs type 2 diabetes, and in patients with and without diabetic complications.

The detail in which we specify the patient population is a double-edged sword. On the one hand, being very specific (middle-aged women with uncomplicated type 2 diabetes) will ensure that the answer we get is applicable to our patients. We may, however, fail to find any studies that restrict themselves to this population. The solution is to start with a specific patient population but be ready to drop specifications to find a relevant article. In this case, we may be ready to drop the "female," "middle-aged," "uncomplicated," and "type 2," in that order. If we suspect that optimal target blood pressure may be similar in diabetic and nondiabetic patients, and it proves absolutely necessary, we might drop the "diabetes."

We may wish to specify that we are interested in the addition of a specific antihypertensive agent. Alternatively, the intervention of interest may be any antihypertensive treatment. Furthermore, a key part of the intervention will be the target for blood pressure control. For instance, we might be interested in knowing whether it makes any difference if our target diastolic blood pressure is less than 80 mm Hg vs less than 90 mm Hg. Another limitation of the initial question formulation is that it fails to specify the criteria by which we will judge the appropriate target for our hypertensive treatment.

Improved (Searchable) Question
A question of THERAPY

- *Patients:* Hypertensive type 2 diabetic patients without diabetic complications.

- *Intervention:* Any antihypertensive agent aiming at a target diastolic blood pressure of 90 mm Hg vs a comparison target of 80 mm Hg.

- *Outcomes:* Stroke, myocardial infarction, cardiovascular death, total mortality.

Example 2: Transient Loss of Consciousness

A 55-year-old man, previously well, although a heavy drinker, presents to the emergency department with an episode of transient loss of consciousness. On the evening of presentation, he had his usual 5 beers and started to climb the stairs at bedtime. The next thing he remembers is being woken by his son, who found him lying near the bottom of the stairs. The patient took about a minute to regain consciousness and remained confused for another 2 minutes. His son did not witness any shaking, and there had not been any incontinence. Physical examination result was unremarkable; the electrocardiogram showed a sinus rhythm with a rate of 80/min and no abnormalities. Glucose, sodium, and other laboratory results were normal.

Initial Question: How extensively should I investigate this patient?

Digging Deeper: The initial question gives us little idea of where to look in the literature for an answer. As it turns out, there is a host of questions that could be helpful in choosing an optimal investigational strategy. We could, for instance, pose a question of differential diagnosis: If we knew the distribution of ultimate diagnoses in such patients, we could choose to investigate the more common and omit investigations targeted at remote possibilities.

Other information that would help us would be the properties of individual diagnostic tests. If an electroencephalogram were extremely accurate for diagnosing a seizure, or a 24-hour Holter monitor for diagnosing arrhythmia, we would be far more inclined to order the tests than if they missed patients with the underlying problems or falsely labeled patients without the problems.

Alternatively, we could ask a question of prognosis. If patients like ours had a benign prognosis, we might be much less eager to investigate extensively than if patients tended to do badly. Finally, the ultimate answer to how intensively we should investigate might come from a randomized trial in which patients similar to this man were allocated to more vs less intensive investigation.

Improved (Searchable) Questions:
A question of DIFFERENTIAL DIAGNOSIS

- *Patients:* Middle-aged patients presenting with transient loss of consciousness.
- *Intervention/Exposure:* Thorough investigation and follow-up.
- *Outcomes:* Frequency of underlying disorders such as vasovagal syncope, seizure, arrhythmia, and transient ischemic attack.

A question of DIAGNOSIS

- *Patients:* Middle-aged patients presenting with transient loss of consciousness.
- *Intervention/Exposure:* Electroencephalogram.
- *Outcomes:* Gold standard investigation (probably long-term follow-up).

A question of PROGNOSIS

- *Patients:* Middle-aged patients presenting with transient loss of consciousness.
- *Intervention/Exposure:* Time.
- *Outcomes:* Morbidity (complicated arrhythmias or seizures, strokes, serious accidents) and mortality in the year after presentation.

A question of THERAPY

- *Patients:* Middle-aged patients presenting with loss of consciousness.

- *Intervention/Exposure:* Comprehensive investigation vs a comparator of minimal investigation.

- *Outcomes:* Morbidity and mortality in the year after presentation.

Example 3: Squamous Cell Carcinoma

A 60-year-old man with a 40-pack-year smoking history presents with hemoptysis. A chest radiograph shows a parenchymal mass with a normal mediastinum, and a fine-needle aspiration of the mass shows squamous cell carcinoma. Aside from hemoptysis, the patient is asymptomatic and physical examination result is entirely normal.

Initial Question: What investigations should we undertake before deciding whether to offer this patient surgery?

Digging Deeper: The key defining features of this patient are his non–small cell carcinoma and the fact that his medical history, physical examination, and chest radiograph show no evidence of intrathoracic or extrathoracic metastatic disease. Alternative investigational strategies address 2 separate issues: Does the patient have occult mediastinal disease, and does he have occult extrathoracic metastatic disease? For this discussion, we will focus on the former issue. Investigational strategies for addressing the possibility of occult mediastinal disease include undertaking a mediastinoscopy or performing a computed tomographic (CT) scan of the chest and proceeding according to the results of this investigation.

What outcomes are we trying to influence in our choice of investigational approach? We would like to prolong the patient's life, but the extent of his underlying tumor is likely to be the major determinant of survival, and our investigations cannot change that. We wish to detect occult mediastinal metastases if they are present because, if the cancer has spread to the mediastinum, resectional surgery is unlikely to benefit the patient. Thus, in the presence of mediastinal disease, patients will usually receive palliative approaches and avoid an unnecessary thoracotomy.

We could frame our structured clinical question in 2 ways. One would be asking about the usefulness of the CT scan for identifying mediastinal disease. More definitive would be to ask a question of therapy: what investigational strategy would yield superior clinical outcomes?

Improved (Searchable) Questions:
A question of DIAGNOSIS

- *Patients:* Newly diagnosed non–small cell lung cancer with no evidence of extrapulmonary metastases.

- *Intervention*: CT scan of the chest.

- *Outcome:* Mediastinal spread at mediastinoscopy.

A question of THERAPY

- *Patients:* Newly diagnosed non–small cell lung cancer with no evidence of extrapulmonary metastases.

- *Intervention*: Mediastinoscopy for all or restricted to those with suspicious lesions on CT scan of the thorax.

- *Outcome:* Unnecessary thoracotomy.

DEFINING THE QUESTION: CONCLUSION

Constructing a searchable question that allows you to use the medical literature to solve problems is no simple matter. It requires a detailed understanding of the clinical issues involved in patient management. The 3 examples in this chapter illustrate that each patient encounter may trigger a number of clinical questions and that you must give careful thought to what you really want to know. Bearing the structure of the question in mind—patient, intervention

3: WHAT IS THE QUESTION? 31

or exposure and control, and outcome—is extremely helpful in arriving at an answerable question. Identifying the type of questions—therapy, harm, differential diagnosis, diagnosis, and prognosis—will further ensure that you are looking for a study with an appropriate design.

Careful definition of the question will provide another benefit: you will be less likely to be misled by a study that addresses a question related to the one in which you are interested, but with 1 or more important differences. For instance, making sure that the study compares experimental treatment to current optimal care may highlight the limitations of trials that use a *placebo* control rather than an alternative active agent. Specifying that you are interested in patient-important outcomes (such as long bone fractures) makes vivid the limitations of studies that focus on *substitute* or *surrogate endpoints* (such as bone density). Specifying that you are primarily interested in avoiding progression to dialysis will make you appropriately wary of a *composite endpoint* of progression to dialysis or doubling of serum creatinine level. You will not reject such studies out of hand, but the careful definition of the question will help you to critically apply the results to your patient care.

A final crucial benefit from careful consideration of the question is that it sets the stage for efficient and effective literature searching to identify and retrieve the best evidence. Chapter 4, Finding the Evidence, uses the components of patient, intervention, and outcome for the questions in this chapter to provide you with the searching tools you will need for effective *evidence-based practice*.

References

1. Yusuf S. Intensive insulin-glucose infusion regimens with long-term or standard glucose control did not differ for reducing mortality in type 2 diabetes mellitus and MI. *ACP J Club.* 2005;143(2):43.
2. Kenealy TAB. Review: mixed signals from trials concerning pharmacological prevention of type 2 diabetes mellitus. *ACP J Club.* 2005;143(2):44.

FINDING THE EVIDENCE

Ann McKibbon, Peter Wyer, Roman Jaeschke,
and Dereck Hunt

IN THIS CHAPTER:

INTRODUCTION

Assessment of knowledge gaps, question formulation, gathering and synthesis of *evidence*, and application of that *evidence* to the care of patients are among the foundations of informed health care. Clinicians frequently use information resources such as textbooks, MEDLINE, and consultation with respected colleagues in gathering evidence. Many information resources exist, and each discipline and subspecialty of medicine has unique information tools and resources. Not all resources, however, provide sound information that can be easily and efficiently accessed. This chapter will help you hone your information-seeking skills and guide you in choosing the best resources for your clinical use.

We begin by describing one way of categorizing resources and then review some of the most useful resources in detail, concentrating on those that are evidence based with high potential for clinical impact. We end the chapter by illustrating searching strategies in several of the databases that can be challenging to use. Our goal is not to discuss all possible choices, but rather to provide a representative sample of the most useful resources and a framework for you to explore different types and classes. Few "best buy" recommendations are in this chapter. A resource's usefulness to you is contingent on many factors, such as your institutional provision of resources, your specialty, your stage of training, and your familiarity with the specific topic of a search. In addition, little evidence exists that compares resources. The American Board of Internal Medicine is studying this issue. They will make their findings public in late 2008.

We will address finding information to answer *background questions* and *foreground questions*, as well as searching related to browsing and keeping up to date.

To start our consideration of external information resources, let us quickly review the distinction between background questions and foreground questions described in the previous chapter (see Chapter 3, What Is the Question?).

Background questions can involve a single fact such as the causative microbiologic agent of Chagas disease, a recommended dose of a drug, or a list of the attributes of the CHARGE syndrome (coloboma of the eye, heart defects, atresia of the choanae, retardation of growth and/or development, genital and/or urinary abnormalities, and ear abnormalities and deafness). Often, they involve much more information such as questions of "What is Gerstmann syndrome?" or "How do I insert a jugular venous central line?"

Foreground questions—targeted questions that provide the evidentiary basis for specific clinical decisions—are best structured using the framework of patient, intervention or exposure, a possible comparison intervention, and *outcomes* of interest: the PICO format. This chapter, and the *Users' Guides* overall, focuses on efficiently finding the best answers to foreground questions.

FOUR CATEGORIES OF INFORMATION SOURCES AND HOW CLINICIANS USE THEM

Table 4-1 summarizes 4 categories of information resources. A fuller description of each category with examples of resources follows.

1. *Systems:* Some information resources provide regularly updated clinical evidence, sometimes integrated with other types of health care information, and provide guidance or recommendations for patient management. Existing systems include PIER (http://pier.acponline.org/index.html), UpTo-Date (http://www.uptodate.com/), *Clinical Evidence* (http://

TABLE 4-1

Categories of Clinical Information Resources

Category	Description	Degree of Evidence Processing	How Many Exist	Ease of Use
Systems	Textbook-like resources that summarize and integrate clinical evidence with other types of information directed at clinical practice decisions/directions	Substantial processing with the integration of evidence and practice—can direct care (give answers) or provide evidence on a clinical action	Few	Very easy
Synopses	Summaries of studies and systematic reviews that include guides or advice for application by expert clinicians	Evidence is externally assessed, with strengths and weaknesses provided for each article/topic	Several thousand	Easy
Summaries	Systematic review of articles and clinical practice guidelines—you assess the information and make decisions	Systematic reviews and high-quality guidelines summarize and present evidence from primary studies; some exemplary guidelines can also be considered synopses	Fewer than 50000	Use may be time consuming and access to full text may require some searching

(*Continued*)

TABLE 4-1

Categories of Clinical Information Resources (*Continued*)

Category	Description	Degree of Evidence Processing	How Many Exist	Ease of Use
Studies	Individual studies (eg, MEDLINE articles)	No processing of evidence at all—individuals must assess and apply	In the millions	Requires the clinician to critically appraise; they are hard to find and may require searching large databases

Derived from Haynes.[1]

www.clinicalevidence.com/ceweb/conditions/index.jsp),
and EBM Guidelines: Evidence-Based Medicine (http://
www3.interscience.wiley.com/cgi-bin/mrwhome/112605734/
HOME).

2. *Synopses:* Preappraised resource journals and products such
   as *ACP Journal Club* (http://www.acpjc.org/) and Info-
   POEMs (http://www.infopoems.com/) serve 2 functions.
   Initially, the articles act as an alerting service to keep
   physicians current on recent advances. When rigorously
   and systematically assembled, the content of such resources
   becomes, over time, a database of important articles. The
   New York Academy of Medicine maintains a list of preappraised resource journals for various disciplines (http://
   www.ebmny.org/journal.html).

3. *Summaries:* The Cochrane Collaboration (http://www.
   cochrane.org/index.htm) provides systematic reviews of
   health care interventions, whereas the Campbell Collaboration provides similar reviews in the social, behavioral, and
   educational arenas (http://www.campbellcollaboration.org/).
   You can also find systematic reviews in MEDLINE and
   other databases. By collecting the evidence on a topic,

systematic reviews become more useful than individual or *primary studies*.

4. *Studies:* Original or primary studies (eg, those stored in MEDLINE). Many studies exist but the information they contain needs evaluation before application to clinical problems.

Clinical practice guidelines illustrate that this classification (like any other) has its limitations: guidelines have aspects of systems and summaries, and sometimes of synopses. For instance, DARE (Database of Abstracts of Reviews of Effects; http://www.york.ac.uk/inst/crd/crddatabases.htm) not only includes reviews themselves but also has elements of guidelines in that expert commentators suggest how clinicians might apply the findings of the reviews.

Clinicians use resources corresponding to all of the above categories to find the information they need during clinical care.[2] Not all resources, however, yield useful answers to clinical questions. Several studies[2-4] show that when clinicians use information resources to answer clinical questions, the resources they choose provide the best evidence only about 50% of the time. Despite this, some evidence suggests that searching for external information improves patient-care processes and may improve health outcomes.[5-8]

SEARCHING THE MEDICAL LITERATURE IS SOMETIMES FUTILE

Consider the following clinical question: In patients with pulmonary embolism, to what extent do those with pulmonary infarction have a poorer *outcome* than those without pulmonary infarction?

Before formulating our search strategy and beginning our literature search to answer this question, we should think about how investigators would differentiate between those with and without infarction. Because no 100% definitive method, short of autopsy, makes this differentiation, our literature search is doomed before we even begin.

This example illustrates that the medical literature will not help you when no feasible study design exists that investigators could use to resolve an issue. Your search will also be futile if no one has taken the time and effort to conduct and publish the necessary study. Before embarking on a search, carefully consider whether the yield is likely to be worth the time expended.

FOUR CRITERIA FOR CHOOSING INFORMATION RESOURCES

Efficient searching involves choosing information sources appropriate for the clinical question—in much the same way you choose diagnostic tests appropriate for your patient's symptoms. The scheme in Table 4-1 offers an initial guideline for making choices. If a fully integrated and reliable resource (a "system" type resource) is likely to address your question, you would be wise to consider it. Depending on the level of detail you need, a *practice guideline* or systematic review, or a well-done synopsis of a guideline or systematic review, could be the next best option. For some questions, you will seek individual studies.

Table 4-2 describes selection criteria that are specific to deciding on an optimal information source. Although most clinicians would like at least 1 comprehensive source of information on which they can rely, the particularities of the question being asked may demand access to a variety of resources.

Soundness of Evidence-Based Approach
An evidence-based information resource will provide access to a representative sample of the highest quality of evidence addressing a clinical question. Evidence-based resources that summarize evidence will explicitly frame their question, conduct a comprehensive search, assess the *validity* of the individual studies, and if appropriate provide a pooled estimate of the impact of the *outcomes* of interest (see Chapter 14, Summarizing the Evidence). Evidence-based resources that provide recommendations will use existing systematic reviews, or conduct their own, to provide best estimates of benefit and *risk* of alternative management strategies for all *patient-important outcomes*.

TABLE 4-2

Selection Criteria for Choosing or Evaluating Resources

Criterion	Description of Criterion
Soundness of evidence-based approach	1. How strong is the commitment to evidence to support inference? 2. How well does the resource indicate the strength of the evidence behind the recommendations or other content? 3. Does the resource provide links for those who wish to view the evidence?
Comprehensiveness and specificity	1. Does the resource cover my discipline or content area adequately? 2. Does it cover questions of the type I am asking (eg, therapy, diagnosis, prognosis, harm)? 3. Does it target my specific area of practice?
Ease of use	1. Does it give me the kind of information I need quickly and consistently?
Availability	1. Is it readily available in all locations in which I would use it? 2. Can I easily afford it?

They then will use an appropriate system to grade recommendations and will make explicit underlying *values and preferences* (see Chapter 15, How to Use a Patient Management Recommendation).

Comprehensiveness and Specificity

An ideal resource will cover most of the questions relevant to your practice—and that is all. Thus, resources limited to your area of practice, such as collections of synopses designed to help you keep up on the latest developments (eg, *Evidence-Based Cardiovascular Medicine*, *Evidence-Based Mental Health*, and *Evidence-Based Oncology*), may serve your needs most efficiently.

Some resources are specific to particular types of questions. For example, Clinical Evidence and Cochrane Database of Systematic Reviews currently restrict themselves to management issues and do not include studies of diagnostic accuracy (although both plan to soon include this material). The databases of the Cochrane Library are confined to *controlled trials* and systematic reviews of such trials.

Ease of Use

Some resources are easy and quick to use. For example, the relatively small size of the *ACP Journal Club* database facilitates searching. The database contains a collection of synopses of the most relevant high-quality studies appearing in approximately 140 journals related to internal medicine. Its excellent search engine further ensures an easy search for anything from viniyoga for low back pain through *meta-analyses* on cholesterol-lowering drugs or breast cancer associated with oral contraceptive use.

MEDLINE is much more challenging to use efficiently because of its size: slightly less than 17 million articles at the start of 2008 (http://www.nlm.nih.gov/bsd/licensee/2008_stats/baseline_med_filecount.html) and growing at the rate of 700 000 articles per year. PubMed, an interface to MEDLINE, is one of the easier ways of using MEDLINE. PubMed is designed for clinicians and includes features such as "Clinical Queries" that limit retrievals to those articles with high probability of being relevant to clinical decisions.

Clinicians may also find the Cochrane reviews challenging. Although you will usually be able to find a relevant Cochrane review quickly when it exists, the reviews are so comprehensive, complex, and variable in the quality of their presentation that they often require considerable time to digest and apply.

Availability

The most trustworthy and efficient resources are frequently expensive. Academic physicians characteristically have access to the online information resources of their medical school or hospital libraries, including the full texts of many journal articles. Physicians in private practice in high–gross domestic product countries may have access to some resources through their professional associations but otherwise may be burdened by the cost of subscriptions. Health professionals in poorer countries may have institutional access through the World Health Organization Health InterNetwork Access to Research Initiative (HINARI) project (http://www.who.int/hinari/en/) or other organizations but otherwise face even greater financial obstacles. Nevertheless, some resources such as PubMed and certain journals (eg, *Canadian Medical Association Journal* and most BioMed Central journals) are free to everyone (http://www.gfmer.ch/Medical_journals/Free_medical.php). Many other journals provide free access to content 6 to 12 months after publication (eg, *BMJ*, *JAMA*, and the *Mayo Proceedings*) or a portion of their contents at the time of publication. *Merck Manual*, an often-used online textbook (http://www.merck.com/mrkshared/mmanual/home.jsp), is also free. However, it largely fails the criterion of being as evidence based in its approach as some of the fee-based resources.

INFORMATION SOURCES THAT DO WELL ON AT LEAST SOME CRITERIA

Tables 4-3 and 4-4 provide brief comparative information concerning examples of resources in each category (systems, synopses, summaries, and studies). Table 4-3 includes those information resources that synthesize data and provide summaries of existing knowledge. For these resources, we include explicit discussions of how evidence is assessed and how this is transmitted to the users of specific information.

Table 4-4 includes those resources that do not synthesize data—they provide access to individual systematic reviews and original studies. We have included some of the major players in each table while trying to include some low-cost (or free) resources for those with limited budgets. The cost of resources is variable, depending on many factors, including individual vs library subscriptions and nationality. We have used US dollars rounded to the nearest $50 and late 2007 pricing for individual subscriptions. At the end of the tables, we offer a narrative description of the individual resources, paying special attention to their purpose and how they are prepared.

TABLE 4-3

Categorization of Representative Examples of Information Resources Readily Available

Category/ Examples of Category	Soundness of Evidence-Based Approach	Comprehensiveness	Ease of Use and Availability/Cost in US Dollars Rounded to the Nearest $50
Textbook-like Resources (Systems)			
Clinical Evidence	Strong	Only therapy; mainly primary care	Easy to use; commercially available; $300 for online and print version
PIER	Strong	Mostly therapy; mainly primary care and internal medicine	Easy to use; commercially available; $100 for PDA version
UpToDate	Strong	Most clinical areas, especially internal medicine and primary care	Easy to use, although searching somewhat lacking; $450 for individuals for their first year, then $350 per year; $10000 plus for libraries
DynaMed	Strong	Most clinical areas, especially internal medicine and primary care	Easy to use; $200 but free if you help in the development
EBM Guidelines	Strong	Most areas of primary-care practice	Internet versions $100; mobile (handheld PC, palm or telephone based) + Internet version $300; print $400; libraries and groups priced individually
Merck Manual	Weak	Covers most clinical areas	Easy to use; free

(*Continued*)

TABLE 4-3

Categorization of Representative Examples of Information Resources Readily Available (*Continued*)

Category/ Examples of Category	Soundness of Evidence-Based Approach	Comprehensiveness	Ease of Use and Availability/Cost in US Dollars Rounded to the Nearest $50
Preappraised (Synopses)			
ACP Journal Club	Strong	Recently published internal medicine studies; covers all categories of studies	Easy to use; $100 for print version
InfoPOEMs	Strong	Recently published family medicine studies; covers all categories of studies	Easy to use; $250
DARE (Database of Abstracts of Reviews of Effects) York, UK	Strong	Covers all disciplines; concentrates on therapy and prevention; summaries of systematic reviews of studies of diagnostic test performance may also be found	Easy to use; free
Bandolier	Strong	Limited coverage for primary-care physicians in the UK	Easy to use; $100 for print version, online free, although a lag time of several months between the two

TABLE 4-4

Information Resources That Provide Access to Systematic Reviews and Original Studies (Weight of the Evidence Applies to Each Study or Review Rather Than to the Total Resource)

Category/ Examples of Categories	Comprehensiveness	Ease of Use/ Availability
Systematic Reviews and Guidelines (Syntheses)		
Systematic reviews	Reviews of use in clinical care are often limited in scope; therefore, one needs to be able to quickly identify whether a relevant article exists	Hard to find and then even harder to get in full text; also need some work to apply the information in the review for clinical care
US National Guidelines Clearinghouse	Comprehensive coverage of US and many other nations' guidelines; often several guidelines on the same topic	Easy to search; one of the strengths of the site is being able to "compare" guidelines on the same topic; free; many full-text guidelines available
Cochrane Database of Systematic Reviews	Covers broad range of disciplines; limited to therapy and prevention	Easy to find a Cochrane review but sometimes difficult to apply because of the depth of coverage; $300 but abstracts free; included in many composite resources such as Ovid
Primary Studies		
MEDLINE	Lots of primary studies across all disciplines and areas of research	Hard to find a specific study and often difficult to use; free through PubMed
Cochrane Controlled Trials Registry (CCTR)	All specialties and all topics for which a controlled trial is relevant (therapy and prevention mainly)	The Cochrane Library includes DARE, Cochrane systematic reviews, and CCTR; $300 for the whole library; the fastest way to determine whether a controlled trial has been published on the topic

(Continued)

TABLE 4-4

Information Resources That Provide Access to Systematic Reviews and Original Studies (Weight of the Evidence Applies to Each Study or Review Rather Than to the Total Resource) (*Continued*)

Category/ Examples of Categories	Comprehensiveness	Ease of Use/ Availability
Primary Studies		
PubMed Clinical Queries	Limits searches to those articles with some possibility of having direct clinical application	Easier to use than MEDLINE because the queries turn MEDLINE into a clinical tool; free
CINAHL	Nursing database costs are high for those not associated with a teaching facility, hospital library	Similar to MEDLINE in that the size introduces problems with being able to search easily and efficiently
Others		
Google	One of the major search engines to the Web—almost everything	Easy to find something, hard to find just what you want and to know the worth and evidence behind the content; fastest way to find high-impact articles that have recently made press and media headlines
SumSearch	One search system for many of the major health databases—one-stop searching; comprehensive	Easy to use; free access
TRIP	A single search system for 150 health databases; one-stop searching; comprehensive; also has 27 specialist subsections (allergy to urology)	Easy to use; free access

(*Continued*)

TABLE 4-4

Information Resources That Provide Access to Systematic Reviews and Original Studies (Weight of the Evidence Applies to Each Study or Review Rather Than to the Total Resource) (*Continued*)

Category/ Examples of Categories	Comprehensiveness	Ease of Use/ Availability
MEDLINEPlus	Comprehensive, with major emphasis on patient/consumer information; some good background information for physicians	Patient information with links to Web sites; free
Individual Web sites	Broad coverage but scattered	Almost unlimited and unknowable information; free

Often, information resources are available in various packages or formats of information (eg, the Internet, on PDAs, as standalone electronic or paper-based resources, and integrated into service packages). The vendor or supplier of the product or a librarian associated with your institution or professional group can help you determine your options for access. We end the chapter by providing search hints for those resources that are potentially useful for a broad range of clinicians but may be challenging to use efficiently.

Textbook-like Resources (Systems)

Clinical Evidence from the *BMJ* Publishing Group (http://www.clinicalevidence.com/ceweb/conditions/index.jsp) covers more than 200 diseases and 2500 treatments and is regularly updated and extended with new topics. Its content draws on published systematic reviews or reviews that the staff completes for authors and is presented in question format (eg, Does regular use of mouthwashes reduce halitosis?). The resource provides the evidence for benefits and *harms* for specific treatments and tells you if the *evidence* is weak or nonexistent (eg, sugar-free gum for halitosis). *Clinical Evidence* has started to begin to address some issues of diagnosis.

PIER is the Physician Information Education and Resource from the American College of Physicians (http://pier.acponline.org/index.html). Its strengths are the direction that it provides for the clinician and the strong evidence-based approach. Authors who are clinical experts receive notification of newly published studies and systematic review articles that have importance to their chapter. Chapters are carefully built around a consistent structure, and all recommendations are tightly linked to the evidence behind the recommendation.

In contrast to *Clinical Evidence*, PIER provides explicit recommendations. Content and evidence are presented using standard methods across diseases and disciplines. The authors of each chapter explicitly state their question, are comprehensive in considering all interventions and patient-important outcomes, assess the validity of individual studies, use a high-quality grading system, and make their values and preference explicit. PIER focuses on treatment, although it does include diagnosis and legal and ethical aspects of health care issues. Its major limitation is lack of comprehensive coverage.

UpToDate is an online textbook that, at least in part because of its ease of use, comprehensiveness, and inclusion of disease-oriented information, is very popular with generalists, specialists, and particularly house staff (http://www.uptodate.com/index.asp). Like PIER, and unlike *Clinical Evidence*, UpToDate provides recommendations (guidelines) for clinicians. It is pricey for libraries, although costs for individuals are similar to those of other information products. Although there is some variation in the extent to which it currently succeeds across topics, UpToDate is committed to structured formulation of questions, identifying an unbiased selection of relevant evidence-based literature on a wide-ranging (though not comprehensive) search, and, in its latest development, using the grades of recommendation, assessment, development, and evaluation (GRADE) system to assess quality of evidence and strength of recommendations.[9] UpToDate explicitly acknowledges the importance of values and preferences in decision making and includes value and preference statements.

DynaMed is a service for primary-care physicians with almost 2000 disease summaries that are updated with information from journal hand-searches and electronic scans of more than 500 journal titles (http://www.dynamicmedical.com/). All information has levels of evidence and grades of recommendations. Although you can obtain DynaMed by subscription or through your library, if you volunteer to help build the resource, you receive free access to the database.

EBM Guidelines is a series of recommendations covering a wide range of topics relevant to primary care. It was originally produced by the Finnish Medical Society with government funding to provide evidence-based guidelines and recommendations for national use. All guidelines are reviewed annually. Recommendations are linked to the evidence, and both the Cochrane and DARE systematic reviews are summarized to produce and maintain a comprehensive collection of treatment and diagnostic guidelines. Recommendations are linked to almost 1000 clinical guidelines and 2500 graded evidence summaries, with more than 350 clinical experts as authors. Images and audio files are also included. Specialists consulting on neighboring specialties may find it of use. It is available in several languages, including English, Finnish, German, Swedish, Russian, Estonian, and Hungarian, with more to follow. Subscription information is at http://www.ebm-guidelines.com.

Merck Manual is available on the Internet at no cost. Unlike UpToDate or *Clinical Evidence*, a systematic consideration of current research does not routinely underlie its recommendations. Strengths include its comprehensiveness, user friendliness, and zero cost (http://www.merck.com/mrkshared/mmanual/home.jsp).

Preappraised Resources (Synopses)

ACP Journal Club, *Evidence-Based Medicine*, and a number of journals modeled on *ACP Journal Club* are available by print subscription or as online publications. The research staff of *ACP Journal Club* read 140 core health care and specialty journals to identify high-quality studies and review articles that have potential for clinical application (those that have strong methods, answer a clinical question, and report data on clinically important outcomes).

From this pool of articles, practicing physicians choose the most clinically important studies with the greatest potential clinical impact. These are then summarized in structured abstracts. A clinical expert comments on methods and provides advice on application of the findings. Only 1 in approximately 150 articles is deemed important enough for abstracting. The online version (current issues and a searchable database of all content) is available from the American College of Physicians or through the Ovid Technologies collection of databases. *ACP Journal Club* is aimed largely at internal medicine and its subspecialties but also includes limited entries relevant to other specialties including pediatrics.

InfoPOEMs is similar to *ACP Journal Club* in that it provides alerting to well-done and important clinical advances and a searching service of its collected articles. Its main focus is family medicine. Clinical staff read more than 100 journals for articles of direct application to common and uncommon diseases and conditions seen by family physicians. The compilation of past issues (searchable database) is called InfoRETRIEVER (http://www.infopoems.com/). Well structured and well presented, all articles have a clinical bottom line for primary-care decisions that users appreciate. Like *ACP Journal Club*, InfoPOEMs is restricted in its scope of practice and to recently published articles. Subscription includes regular e-mail notification of new evidence, as well as downloading to individual computers and ongoing Web access.

Bandolier provides a summary service for the National Health Service in the United Kingdom that is also available worldwide (http://www.jr2.ox.ac.uk/bandolier/). It covers selected clinical topics over a broad range of disciplines and combines a review of clinical evidence with clinical commentary and recommendations.

The New York Academy of Medicine Web site (http://www.ebmny.org/journal.html) provides a list of these preappraised resources (synopses) including specialty-specific journals modeled on *ACP Journal Club*. Non-English examples of preappraised resources exist. For example, Medycyna Praktyczna is published in Polish (http://www.mp.pl). *Evidence-Based Medicine*, the synoptic journal for primary-care physicians and internists published by the BMJ Publishing Group (http://ebm. bmjjournals.com/), is also translated into French (http://www. ebm-journal.presse.fr/) and Italian (http://www.infomedica.com/ebm.htm).

Systematic Reviews and Guidelines (Summaries)

Cochrane Database of Systematic Reviews, built and maintained by the Cochrane Collaboration, contains systematic reviews that cover almost all health care interventions (therapy and prevention) (http://www3. interscience.wiley.com/cgi-bin/mrwhome/106568753/HOME). As of the 2008 Issue 1, 3385 reviews had been completed, with an additional 1786 posted protocols of reviews in progress. Each review is extremely comprehensive—to a fault. The Cochrane reviews are available in many forms and from various vendors (eg, in Ovid and PubMed, as well as standalone and Web versions from Wiley InterScience). Searching is easy, although some systems are easier to use than others. Abstracts are free, but the full reviews require a subscription or institutional source. Some countries such as the United Kingdom, Australia, New Zealand, and Iceland have country-wide access provided by government funding, and some lower-GDP countries have been granted free access (http://www3.interscience.wiley.com/cgi-bin/mrwhome/106568753/DoYouAlreadyHaveAccess.html). Most academic and large hospital libraries provide access to the full text of the Cochrane reviews.

DARE (Database of Abstracts of Reviews of Effects) is a free database of critically appraised summaries of non-Cochrane systematic reviews in a broad range of health topics and disciplines (http://www.york.ac.uk/inst/crd/crddatabases.htm#DARE). It is a standalone Web-based resource and is also included in the Cochrane Library. DARE includes more systematic reviews than does Cochrane, but the DARE reviews are not as comprehensive—more than 600 reviews are added annually. DARE is easy and fast to search, and the developers pay attention to the strength of the evidence of each review they summarize. The DARE summaries of others' reviews may be particularly useful to clinicians who do not have either the time to appraise or electronic access to the full text of the original reviews—this feature allows some people to suggest that DARE can be categorized as a synopses resource.

Clinical practice guidelines that are strongly evidence based provide helpful direction for decision making by health professionals. The US National Guidelines Clearinghouse database includes the full text of many US and international guidelines on almost all conceivable topics (http://www.guideline.gov/). The Web site includes thousands of guidelines and provides systematic summaries of more than 2200. Searching is easy, although initial retrievals are often relatively large. The site allows comparison of several guidelines on the computer screen at the same time by checking the guidelines you want, adding them to your collection, and comparing the checked guidelines. The resulting information includes a side-by-side comparison of the components of the guideline such as methods of searching the literature and specification of their making values and preferences explicit (see Chapter 15, How to Use a Patient Management Recommendation). Other international guidelines can be found at the UK National Library for Health (http://libraries.nelh.nhs.uk/guidelinesFinder/default.asp?page=INTER). The Ontario Medical Association goes one step further in the evaluation process. They provide a collection of preappraised guidelines that meet strict quality criteria (http://www.gacguidelines.ca/).

Many systematic reviews are included in MEDLINE and other large databases. The systematic reviews are often difficult to retrieve from these databases because of the volume of other citations.

Original/Primary Studies (Studies)

Millions of primary studies exist, and processing of the evidence takes time and effort. Because systems, synopses, and summaries conduct much of this processing, we recommend using original studies in clinical care only when you cannot find the answers to your questions elsewhere. If you do need to retrieve original studies, you will likely use the following large bibliographic databases to aid your retrieval.

MEDLINE is the premier database of health care research and practice. Many of the more traditional methods of access to the MEDLINE articles (eg, Ovid Technologies; http://www.ovid.com/

site/index.jsp?top=1) are designed to facilitate complex search strategies such as those done by medical librarians. You have many options for obtaining access to MEDLINE (http://www.diabetesmonitor.com/ database.htm), although most clinicians use Ovid (through their institutions) or PubMed.

PubMed Clinical Queries (http://www.ncbi.nlm.nih.gov/entrez/ query/static/clinical.shtml) function so that your searching is restricted to a "virtual" database of the studies in MEDLINE that are likely to have direct clinical application. PubMed also can search the whole MEDLINE database.

CINAHL (Cumulative Index to Nursing and Allied Health Literature; http://www.cinahl.com/) database is independent of MEDLINE and is the premier nursing and allied health database. Clinicians of all backgrounds may find it useful to search for articles on *quality of care* and *quality improvement*. It is also rich in *qualitative research*. Emergency physicians may use it as a source for issues relevant to prehospital emergency care. As with other large databases, multiple access routes are available (http://www. cinahl.com/ prodsvcs/prodsvcs.htm).

EMBASE (http://www.elsevier.com/wps/find/bibliographic databasedescription.cws_home/523328/description#description) is a large European database (more than 11 million citations) that is similar to MEDLINE in scope and content, with strengths in drugs and allied health disciplines. Clinicians are unlikely to use EMBASE because of its limited availability—major research institutions rather than hospitals or smaller organizations are the most common suppliers of access based on cost considerations. Up to 70% of citations in EMBASE are not included in MEDLINE.

Cochrane Controlled Trials Registry, part of the Cochrane Library (http://www.cochrane.org/reviews/clibintro.htm), is the largest electronic compilation of controlled trials in existence (527 885 citations as of 2008, Issue 1) and is available as part of a subscription to the Cochrane Library or several Ovid Evidence-Based Medicine Review packages of databases (http://www.ovid.com/site/catalog/DataBase/ 904.jsp?top=2&mid=3&bottom=7&subsection=10). Their registry of original trials is a companion database to the Cochrane systematic reviews database. This registry is built from large databases, including

MEDLINE and EMBASE, as well as other sources used by the review groups within the Cochrane Collaboration, including hand-searches of most major health care journals. The trials registry is the fastest, most reliable method of determining whether a controlled trial has been published on any topic.

Alerting or Updating Services

Electronic communication (ie, e-mail) is an excellent method of keeping clinicians abreast of evidence in newly published studies and systematic reviews. You can easily receive the table of contents of journals or newly published articles on a specific topic or subscribe to a service that notifies you of advances across many journals. PubMed, through its My NCBI service (http://www.ncbi.nlm.nih.gov/books/bv.fcgi?rid=helpPubMed.section.PubMedhelp.My_NCBI), allows you to establish a search that will automatically e-mail you citations of newly published articles based on content (eg, asthma in adolescents) or journal titles. The Chinese University of Hong Kong maintains a Web site with links to sign up for e-mail alerts from all major journal publishers (http://www.lib.cuhk.edu.hk/information/publisher.htm).

Bmjupdates+ is a free alerting service to newly published studies and systematic reviews from 140 journals (http://bmjupdates.mcmaster.ca/index.asp). You choose the frequency with which you want to receive e-mail notifications, choose the disciplines in which you are interested, and set the score level on clinical relevance and newsworthiness as determined by peer raters in multiple disciplines.

InfoPOEMs (http://www.infopoems.com/) also provides e-mail alerts to new clinical evidence in studies and systematic reviews. Each alert includes a clinical bottom line on the application of the findings.

Journal Watch Online is another alerting service (http://www.jwatch.org/issues_by_date.shtml) with a broad coverage of new evidence. *The New England Journal of Medicine* produces this service with the aim of keeping clinicians up to date on the most important research in the general medical literature. Journal Watch provides nonstructured summaries and commentaries on articles it identifies but does not use a quality filter or structured critical appraisal of the sort embodied in the resources described above under synopses.

Other Resources

Many search engines exist for the Internet, of which Google (http://
www.google.com/) is the most popular, followed by Ask (formerly
Ask Jeeves) (http://www.ask.com/), MSN (http://www.msn.com/),
and Yahoo (http://www.yahoo.com/). Search engines either send
out electronic "spiders" that "crawl" the Web to index material for
later retrieval or rely on human indexing of sites. Search Engine
Watch maintains a list of important and heavily used services (http://
searchenginewatch.com/links/article.php/2156221) and rates usefulness of each. Almost limitless amounts of information are available
on the Internet. Characteristically, one finds information from
unsubstantiated or nonscientifically supervised sources freely inter-
spersed with references to articles in peer-reviewed biomedical
journals.

Internet searchers should understand that they are not searching
a defined database but rather are surfing the constantly shifting seas
of electronic communications. The material that is supported by
evidence may not float to the surface at any particular time. On the
other hand, an Internet search may constitute the fastest way of
tracking down an article that has attracted media attention shortly
after its release and during the period in which it has not yet been
indexed by MEDLINE or will not likely be indexed.

Google Scholar (http://scholar.google.com/) is a service that
provides Google-like searching of scholarly information (eg,
articles, dissertations, books, abstracts, and full text from publishers). MEDLINE is included (although it may be up to a year
out of date). You have access to ranked material (most important
and not necessarily the newest information first) and to other
documents that cite an important item you have identified.
Google Scholar has a complex searching system, and the Help
feature is actually quite helpful (http://scholar.google.com/intl/
en/scholar/help.html).

Search engines that retrieve and combine results from multiple search engines (metasearch engines) also exist (http://search
enginewatch.com/links/article.php/2156241):

- **SumSearch** is a medical metasearch engine. By using it, you
  can search multiple medical databases with 1 entry of

search terms (http://sumsearch.uthscsa.edu/). For example, the entry of 1 word, "bedrest," provided grouped links to 27 entries in Wikipedia, 21 guidelines (US National Guidelines Clearinghouse), 18 broad or narrative reviews (good to answer background questions), 1 DARE or Cochrane systematic review, 87 other systematic reviews from PubMed, and 59 original studies covering therapy and etiology studies from PubMed Clinical Queries. In contrast, Google retrieves approximately 588 000 entries on "bedrest" and the items are not grouped by source or like items for easier access.

- **TRIP** is similar to SumSearch in that it searches multiple databases and other strongly evidence-based resources with just 1 entry of your term or terms (http://www.trip database.com/). TRIP currently searches more than 150 databases and related resources. It is rich in systematic reviews, clinical practice guidelines (US, UK, Canadian, Australian, and New Zealand national collections), clinical questions and answers, and medical images. It also has a substantial collection of patient information resources, as well as critical appraisal topics (CATs). It harnesses the PubMed Clinical Queries in its searching and includes links to the bmjupdates+ to enable a more clinically relevant retrieval set of documents. TRIP was once a fee-based system but is now free. It has 27 specialist mini-TRIP systems based on health care content (allergy to urology) early in 2008.

MEDLINEPlus is the premier site for Web links to health information on the Internet. The US National Library of Medicine provides this free service, which is designed to provide high-quality and important health information to patients and families. The staff members provide access to Web sites that meet preestablished quality criteria. Some information is likely useful to clinicians, especially in areas in which they are not experts. Many clinicians feel confident sending their patients to MEDLINEPlus for consumer/patient information (http://medlineplus.gov/).

Format

Information resources are available in many formats: paper, stand-alone computer installations (eg, CD-ROM disks), or via the Internet. The handheld computer is becoming a major player in providing information resources quickly and at the site of care. We have not included a primer on how to choose handhelds or information resources for them. Peers, commercial sites, or the handhelds themselves are the best sources of determining if handheld devices are the vehicle for providing you with information resources.

ADDRESSING EXAMPLE QUESTIONS

The rest of this chapter provides searching tips for question types and specific information resources. We concentrate on resources that are challenging to use effectively and that are readily available.

Background Questions

Most background questions are often best answered by standard textbooks such as *Harrison's Principles of Internal Medicine*, *Nelson Textbook of Pediatrics*, *Benson's Current Obstetric and Gynecological Diagnoses and Treatments*, and *Lawrence's Essentials of General Surgery* or innovative electronic texts such as UpToDate. To provide faster searching for background questions, some companies also group collections of textbooks together to be searched in tandem. Two major collections of medical texts are MDConsult (http://www.mdconsult.com/offers/standard.html) and Stat!Ref (http://www.statref.com/). These collections often include other resources besides textbooks.

Textbooks and other resources classified as systems are often easy to search. Most of them rely on entry of a single concept such as a disease or diagnostic test that leads you to various categories or chapters. The Internet may also be very useful for background questions.

Foreground Questions

The most efficient sources of information for foreground questions are resources that are classified in the information categories of systems and synopses.

Searching in Systems and Synopses-Based Resources (Small Resources)

You can search small-sized resources using common words or phrases such as diseases or conditions and categories such as therapy or prognosis—their size makes them easy and efficient to search. For example, in *ACP Journal Club*, all of the 9 "house dust mite" articles can be found by putting in only "mites" as a searching word (Ovid MEDLINE and PubMed have approximately 10 000 articles on mites). Usually, some simple experimentation with a new system or a few tips from fellow users are sufficient for getting started. Continued experience with the resource usually hones searching skills.

Searching for Synopses and Summaries (Moderately Sized Resources)

As a resource grows, it becomes more difficult to use effectively—single words or simple phrases retrieve too much information. Synopses and summary resources are usually resources that are larger than the systems (textbook-like resources) but far smaller than resources that include studies (eg, MEDLINE). Simple terms and phrases with some category choices are sufficient for smaller resources, but designing effective searching strategies with these larger information resources requires more attention.

The same or similar search strategy may perform differently, depending on the route of access to a particular database. For example, the standalone version of Cochrane systematic reviews by the electronic publisher Wiley InterScience has a search engine that often searches for all occurrences of your search terms across the full information in the database. This method can retrieve large sets of citations, many of which are not relevant but are retrieved because of single occurrences of the search terms.

The Ovid search engine for the same database performs differently. Ovid Technologies is a major resource in providing information to clinicians. Ovid provides access to a large selection of databases, including MEDLINE and the Cochrane Library. Its strength is its comprehensive collection of resources that are accessed using the same searching mechanisms. The drawback of this approach is that because of the size of some of the resources, the searching system is complex, requiring a relatively steep learning curve. Ovid searching is more complex and often more parsimonious. For example, the search of the Cochrane Database of Systematic Reviews using the Ovid interface yields 31 reviews, whereas the Wiley InterScience database yields 42 reviews, even though both systems search for the phrase "patient adherence."

Most resources beyond very small products have tutorials and searching tips, and medical librarians are often available to help you learn how to use a system individually or in a class session.

Searching for Summaries and Primary Studies Using PubMed

If (and only if) resources similar to the ones described above fail to provide an answer to your clinical questions, you then can move to one of the large databases such as MEDLINE. One of the most available systems is PubMed. The US National Library of Medicine has done substantial work to develop the PubMed search interface to the MEDLINE database so that PubMed is easy for clinicians to use effectively. PubMed is free and more than 70 million searches are done each month (http://www.nlm.nih.gov/pubs/factsheets/PubMed.html). The makers of PubMed have developed a useful and comprehensive tutorial (http://www.nlm.nih.gov/bsd/PubMed_tutorial/m2001.html) that can complement trial-and-error learning.

Because PubMed is a useful resource across disciplines and is readily available, we will show you some simple tips and techniques. Our demonstration is designed to equip the reader with a basic orientation. Many clinicians in search of relatively high-quality studies pertaining to a specific question find it expedient to bypass most of this system and to go directly to the Clinical Queries function, which we describe below. To facilitate the effectiveness of these demonstrations, we recommend that you call up PubMed on your own browser and "follow along" by performing the steps yourself as we describe them.

Simple Searching Using Phrases (Natural Language)

Like many other information resources such as Google, PubMed has a single searching box. Just type in a sentence or series of phrases that represent exactly what you are searching. The choice of terms to use will be easy if you have developed questions using the PICO format: patients, intervention, comparison, and outcome. PubMed uses Google spell checker and is programmed to do the work of finding synonyms for your terms—just put in 1 phrase or word per PICO concept. Generally, if you use 3 or more concepts, your retrieval will be limited to a reasonable-sized retrieval. No matter how effective your searching skills, however, your search retrievals will almost inevitably include some citations that are not on topic.

One often successful method to enrich your search retrieval is to click on the Related Articles button to the right of the article in which you are most interested. PubMed will then search for articles it thinks are related to yours. If your initial searching finds an article that is an exact match to your topic, the Related Articles feature is often fruitful to identify more citations.

To show you how these approaches to searching can work, see figures in the text. We started with a PICO question (Table 4-5) looking at determining the ideal gestational age for a term twin pregnancy in a 35-year-old woman who wants to know whether a planned cesarean section or planned vaginal delivery is associated with improved outcomes, specifically, mortality.

TABLE 4-5

PICO and Determination of Searching Terms

PICO	Element	Search Terms for PubMed
P(atient)	Term twin pregnancy	Term twin pregnancy
I(ntervention)	Planned cesarean section	Planned C–section
C(omparison)	Planned vaginal delivery	Vaginal delivery
O(utcome)	Infant mortality	Mortality

We entered the 4 sets of searching terms in January 2008 (term twin pregnancy, planned C-section, vaginal delivery, and mortality) in the PubMed searching box and only found 3 articles (Figure 4-1). The second one, by Smith et al,[10] looks like a very good match to our question. This retrieval set is small and the question of cesarean section or vaginal delivery for twins fairly common; therefore, many more studies have probably addressed this question. Rather than selecting another set of terms and trying again, you can click on the Related Articles link in Figure 4-1. This retrieval is now 1301 articles (Figure 4-2). These are too many, but the search is still useful because the articles are listed in rank order of perceived importance—you only need to scan down the list until you have the information you need or find another citation that you want to check for related articles. This Related Articles method of searching

FIGURE 4-1

PubMed Retrieval Using a Set of Phrases

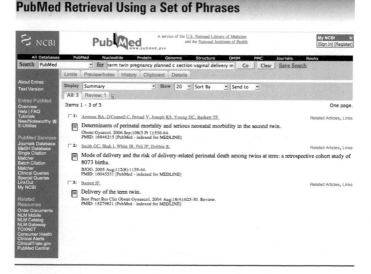

Note the Related Articles links at the right of the citations.

Reproduced with permission of the U.S. National Library of Medicine (NLM) and PubMed.

FIGURE 4-2

Retrieval Based on the Related Articles Link, Going From 3 Citations to Many More Returned in "Importance" Order

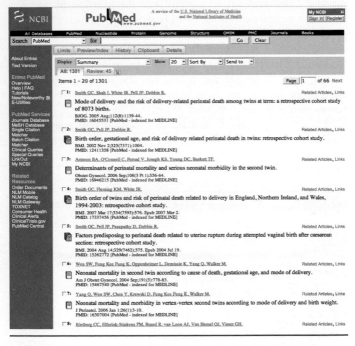

Reproduced with permission of the U.S. National Library of Medicine (NLM) and PubMed.

is very quick and removes the necessity of finding precise searching terms. If you do not like your results, just quickly switch to another set of searching phrases and start the cycle again.

You can also see the related articles as you go through a list of citations. For example, if you were looking for studies that used children's drawings in the diagnosis of migraine headache and retrieved a set of citations that looked interesting, you can ask for the display format to be "AbstractPlus" (Figure 4-3). You will obtain the view below. The main article shows that children's drawings are useful starting at 4 years of age for helping with the diagnosis of migraine. The first related article is an update of the study that shows that the same drawing mechanism can provide data that can plot the success or failure of the treatment of the children's migraines.

FIGURE 4-3

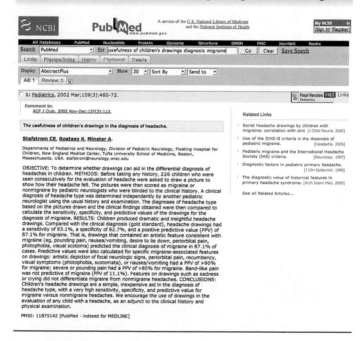

Diagnosis of Migraine in Children by Using Their Drawings

Article presented with links to related articles.

In PubMed, or other systems, you are not limited to phrases that could be in the title or abstract alone. The search in the screen below is one that is set to retrieve an article that we know already exists in *CMAJ*. Belanger studied the timing of infant cereal feeding and the risk for celiac disease. We used the terms "belanger cmaj timing" in Figure 4-4. Note the full-text icon—all articles in *CMAJ* are freely available in full text, and you can get to the whole article directly from a PubMed citation.

Articles that are available in full text have symbols providing this access either at the publisher's site or at PubMed Central. These full-text links are available for several hundred journal titles, and their numbers are increasing. To add to the number of full-text articles to which you have access, some hospital and university libraries have installed links from their collection of full-text journals into PubMed. To access the version of PubMed that is customized for your library and its collection of online journals, check with your librarian to see if this feature is available to you and how best to access it.

FIGURE 4-4

Searching for a Known Article and Notice of Full-Text Availability

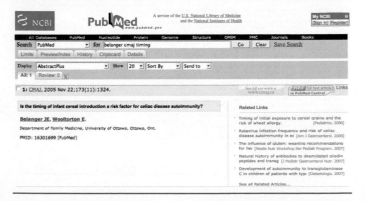

Limits

You can limit your retrieval in PubMed by using all sorts of aspects of individual articles (eg, year of publication, sex of participants, English language, and article type such as a randomized controlled trial [RCT] or meta-analysis). We will look at the function of the limits button in Figure 4-5, as well as describe the ability of PubMed to "understand" your search terms. In the search, we wanted to identify meta-analyses of nursing clinics to reduce hospitalizations in elderly patients with congestive heart failure. The PICO representation of the question follows in Table 4-6. In this case, we are dealing with a patient population rather than a patient—both fit into the PICO format.

Taking advantage of PubMed's ability to recognize alternate searching terms, we limited our typing by entering "heart failure nursing hospitalization" in the search box and clicking on limits for meta-analysis, human participants, participants who are more than 65 years of age, English language, and articles with abstracts (a technique to retrieve more studies and fewer letters and editorials) (Figure 4-5). PubMed automatically translated our search into the strategy in Table 4-7. Note that the concept of hospitalization is searched using US and UK spellings. Note also that this translation of terms does not always work, because we not only got the aspect of using nurses to improve care but also got articles on breast

TABLE 4-6

PICO and Determination of Searching Terms

PICO	Element	Search Terms for PubMed
P(atient/opulation)	Elderly patients with heart failure	Limit by age to > 65 y heart failure
I(ntervention)	Nurse-led clinics	Nursing
C(omparison)	Any	[Nothing—leave concept out]
O(utcome)	Hospital admission	Hospitalization
Other concepts	Meta-analysis	Limit to meta-analysis

FIGURE 4-5

PubMed Searching Showing Limits

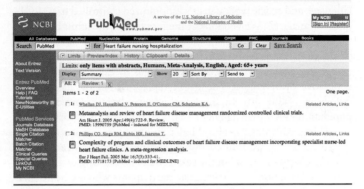

Reproduced with permission of the U.S. National Library of Medicine (NLM) and PubMed.

feeding. Because we added in the geriatric age limit, the breast feeding aspect will likely not complicate our retrieval.

Text word means any occurrence of the word or phrase in the title or abstract of the article; MeSH terms are medical subject headings (controlled vocabulary) that indexes apply to all MEDLINE articles.

TABLE 4-7

PubMed Translation of Concepts into Searching Terms and Strategies

Heart failure	"heart failure" [Text Word] or "heart failure" [MeSH Terms]
Hospitalization	"hospitalization" [Text Word] or "hospitalisation" [Text Word] or "hospitalization" [MeSH Terms]
Nursing	"nursing" [Subheading] or "nursing" [MeSH Terms] or ("breast feeding" [Text Word]) or "breast feeding" [MeSH Terms] or "nursing" [Text Word]
Geriatrics	"aged" [MeSH Terms]
Humans	"humans" [MeSH Terms]

Clinical Queries are available in PubMed, as well as Ovid, and are used by many clinicians to make their MEDLINE searching faster and more efficient for clinical topics. The "path" to Clinical Queries is on the left-hand side of the screen within the blue bar (see Figure 4-5). The screen shots in Figures 4-6 to 4-8 show how one would progress through several screens, looking for high-quality clinical studies assessing the mortality related to binge drinking. The PICO question ("In adults, is binge drinking compared with nonbinge drinking associated with an increase in mortality?") with search terms is included in Table 4-8.

Figure 4-6 shows a search for binge drinking only: it retrieves more than 1100 articles. Adding the Clinical Queries limit for etiology with a broad search (sensitive search) brings the total down to 796—still too high (Figure 4-7). What the clinical queries do in practice is to take a set of search terms that have proven effective at retrieving high-quality clinical articles that have the potential to be important to questions related to

FIGURE 4-6

Binge Drinking Retrievals From All of MEDLINE

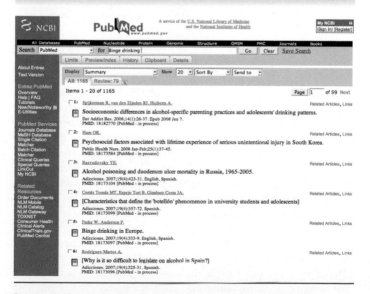

FIGURE 4-7

Clinical Queries Search for Binge Drinking: Broad-Based Etiology/Harm Search

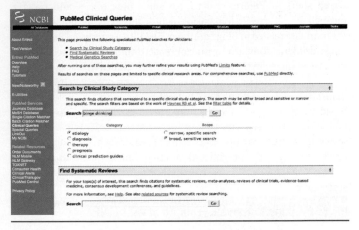

Reproduced with permission of the U.S. National Library of Medicine (NLM) and PubMed.

therapy, diagnosis, etc. You then add your content, in this case binge drinking, and PubMed adds in the appropriate methods terms. For a broad etiology search, these terms are (risk *[Title/Abstract] OR risk *[MeSH:noexp] OR risk *[MeSH:noexp] OR cohort studies [MeSH Terms] OR group*[Text Word]). (The asterisk [*] denotes truncation—picking up multiple endings for the term. The noexp indicates that the system is not picking up terms related but not equivalent to the term in question.) You can see the start of this search strategy string in the searching box of Figure 4-8. Switching to the narrow clinical queries search for etiology (specific search) brings the number of retrieved studies down to approximately 100 citations. Figures 4-9 and 4-10 show you how to "take control" of the searching process and do some of your own manipulation.

By clicking on the "history" tab, you can get to a list of the search statements that you have used in your most recent search session (Figure 4-9). For our search, the statement number 9 is the search that is binge-drinking limited by using the broad clinical category

FIGURE 4-8

Search Retrieval Using the Broad Etiology Hedge

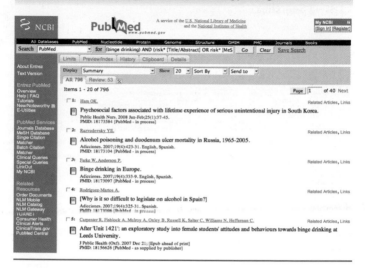

Reproduced with permission of the U.S. National Library of Medicine (NLM) and PubMed.

search for etiology. (If you are following along, your statement number is likely different.) The retrieval for search statement 9 is substantial, and we have not added the concept of "mortality." We

TABLE 4-8

PICO and Determination of Searching Terms

PICO	Element	Search Terms for PubMed
P(atient)	Adults	[Leave blank]
I(ntervention/exposure)	Binge drinking	Binge drinking
C(omparison)	No binge drinking	[Leave blank]
O(utcome)	Mortality	Mortality

FIGURE 4-9

Taking Control of PubMed and Adding Terms of Your Choice to Existing Searches

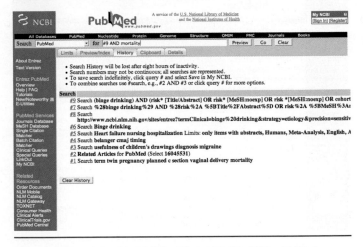

Reproduced with permission of the U.S. National Library of Medicine (NLM) and PubMed.

could do this in several ways. However, for this example, we work with our existing search statements. We want to combine our etiology search on binge drinking with mortality. In the search box at the top of the page, we type in "#9" and combine it with the term "mortality"—note that you can use "AND" or "and" (#9 AND mortality). ANDing in the term "mortality" brings retrieval down to 83 citations of mortality associated with binge drinking, using the etiology clinical queries filter.

Searching for Summaries and Primary Studies Using Other Large Information Resources

The large databases such as MEDLINE, CINAHL, PsycINFO, and EMBASE provide challenges to clinicians wanting to find information directly applicable to clinical care. The size of the database and the relatively few important and relevant studies that are buried within the large volume of literature make the searching complex. Although a few

FIGURE 4-10

Retrieval of ANDing a Word to Previous Searches

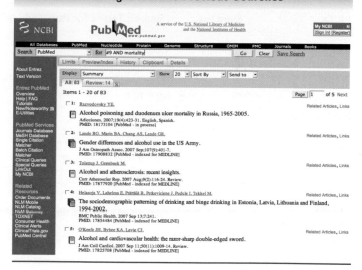

Reproduced with permission of the U.S. National Library of Medicine (NLM) and PubMed.

initial tips followed by trial-and-error practice should allow you to become proficient in doing simple searches, comprehensive searches aiming at high accuracy require the expertise of a research librarian.

Many libraries are equipped with a customized collection of databases and services from Ovid Technologies. Ovid provides a single front-end search and links across databases and services to full texts of articles available to that library system. To show some of the power and complexity of searching using Ovid, we have entered a search in Ovid format designed to look for studies of using either oral or intravenous antibiotics in a 28-year-old male intravenous drug user with endocarditis. The PICO format of the question is shown in Table 4-9.

In Ovid searching, one builds searches idea by idea (Figure 4-11). To start this building process, our first search concept is endocarditis—entering the term and checking it in the list of preferred terminology MeSH shows that, between 1996 and 2008, 5726 articles include information on endocarditis. We have asked the system to

TABLE 4-9

PICO and Determination of Searching Terms

PICO	Element	Search Terms for PubMed
P(atient)	IV drug user	Substance abuse; intravenous
	Endocarditis	Endocarditis
	Adult	Limit to adults (18-44 y)
I(ntervention)	Antibiotics	Antibiotics
	Oral	Administration; oral
C(omparison)	Antibiotics	[Leave blank]—already have it
	Intravenous	Infusions, parenteral
O(utcome)	Any	[Leave blank]

automatically search for all aspects of a topic—this "explode" feature allows for gathering together general aspects of endocarditis and bacterial endocarditis. Using the same approach during the same period, 5679 articles deal with some aspect of intravenous substance abuse, more than 100 000 articles on any antibiotic, almost 40 000 on oral administration of drugs, and more than 25 000 on parenteral infusions. The explosion of parenteral infusions picks up the intravenous infusions, a closer approximation of what we are looking for. We combine the sets and identify only 1 citation that includes all of our concepts. We will stop here, but for illustration purposes, we could also limit to adults, humans, and a clinical query–sensitive search for high-quality therapy articles. We could have also limited on other aspects of retrieval such as English language or articles with abstracts. The retrieved citation is a RCT reported in 1996.[11]

Miscellaneous Searching Issues

We did not cover many aspects of finding information such as looking for health-related statistics. The Web pages of the Univer-

FIGURE 4-11

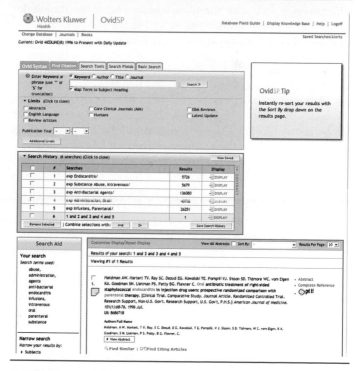

Ovid Searching in MEDLINE Showing a Complex Multistep Search

sity of Michigan (http://www.lib.umich.edu/govdocs/stats.html), the Centers for Disease Control and Prevention, National Center for Health Statistics (http://www.cdc.gov/nchs/), and the National Library of Medicine (http://www.nlm.nih.gov/services/statistics.html) are good places to start looking for international, national, and local statistics on mortality, morbidity, utilization, education, and human resource requirements. We also did not cover searching for some areas of content (eg, *economic evaluation*, *clinical prediction rules*, disease *prevalence*, health services, and qualitative studies). If you want to expand your searching skills in these and other areas, check with the librarians in your organization for individual or group instruction, as well as the searching tips and examples that accompany the scenario at the start of each chapter in this book.

You may also want to develop your own customized resources in specific content areas. Many practitioners find it convenient to compile their own summaries of evidence on topics of particular interest for easy access in the course of teaching and patient care. Such resources may take advantage of institutional informatics capabilities or of options such as the Catmaker, developed by the Centre for Evidence-Based Medicine (http://www.cebm.net/catmaker.asp). The Evidence-Based Emergency Medicine Working Group at the New York Academy of Medicine offers the Journal Club Storage Bank (http://ebem.org/jcb/journalclubbank.html) to emergency teachers and practitioners as an online repository of evidence summaries. Individuals may post their own summaries for easy retrieval. It is password protected to prevent its contents from being misconstrued as electronic publications for external use.[12]

CONCLUSION

In this chapter, we looked briefly at many, but by no means all, potential information resources. We encourage you to consider updating your information tools and develop effective methods of finding the evidence you need in practice. We urge you to use strongly evidence-based resources appropriate for your discipline. Most efficient searching involves seeking information from some of the textbook-like systems first, moving to synopses and summaries of evidence (systematic reviews and clinical practice guidelines) next, and then going to the large bibliographic databases only if required.

Acknowledgments

Conflict of interest statement: Ann McKibbon, Dereck Hunt, and Roman Jaeschke have worked with *ACP Journal Club*; Ann McKibbon received salary support. Roman Jaeschke continues this work. Roman Jaeschke has also researched the use of UpToDate and is an external consultant for this resource. Ann McKibbon and Roman Jaeschke have written Cochrane systematic reviews. Ann McKibbon helped develop PubMed Clinical Queries and bmjupdates+. Peter Wyer is part of the Evidence-Based Emergency Medicine Working Group at the New York Academy of Medicine, which offers the Journal Club Storage Bank. None of the authors will gain personally or financially from the use of any of the resources listed in this chapter.

References

1. Haynes RB. Of studies, syntheses, synopses, and systems: the "4S" evolution of services for finding current best evidence. *ACP J Club*. 2001;134(2):A11-A13.

2. McKibbon KA, Fridsma DB. Effectiveness of clinician-selected electronic information resources for answering primary care physicians' information needs. *JAMA*. 2006;13(6):653-659.

3. Hersh WR, Crabtree MK, Hickman DH, et al. Factors associated with success in searching MEDLINE and applying evidence to answer clinical questions. *J Am Med Inform Assoc*. 2002;9(3):283-293.

4. Westbrook JI, Coirea WE, Gosling AS. Do online information retrieval systems help experienced clinicians answer clinical questions? *JAMA*. 2005;12(3):315-321.

5. Schaafsma F, Verbeek J, Hulshof C, van Dijk F. Caution required when relying on a colleague's advice: a comparison between professional advice and evidence from the literature. *BMC Health Serv Res*. 2005; 5:59.

6. Lindberg D, Siegel ER, Rapp BA, Wallingford KT, Wilson SR. Use of MEDLINE by physicians for clinical problem solving. *JAMA*. 1993;269(24):3124-3129.

7. Klein MS, Ross FV, Adams DL, Gilbert CM. Effect of online literature searching on length of stay and patient care costs. *Acad Med*. 1994; 69(6):489-495.

8. Pluye P, Grad RM, Dunikowski LG, Stephenson R. Impact of clinical information-retrieval technology on physicians: a literature reviews of quantitative, qualitative and mixed methods studies. *Int J Med Inform*. 2005;74(9):745-768.

9. Schünemann HJ, Jaeschke R, Cook DJ, et al; for ATS Documents Development and Implementation Committee. An official ATS statement: grading the quality of evidence and strength of recommendations in ATS guidelines and recommendations. *Am J Respir Crit Care Med*. 2006; 174(5):605-614.

10. Smith CS, Pell JP, Cameron AD, Dobbie R. Mode of delivery and the risk of delivery-related perinatal death among twins at term: a retrospective cohort study of 8073 births. *BJOG*. 2005;112(8):1139-1144.

11. Heldman AW, Hartert TV, Ray SC, et al. Oral antibiotic treatment of right-sided staphylococcal endocarditis in injection drug users: prospective randomized comparison with parenteral therapy. *Am J Med*. 1996; 101(1):68-76.

12. Yeh B, Wyer PC. Bringing Journal Club to the bedside: a hands-on demonstration of an on-line repository allowing electronic storage and point-of-care retrieval of journal club exercises for emergency medicine residency programs [abstract 349]. *Acad Emerg Med*. 1999;6(5):487.

WHY STUDY RESULTS MISLEAD: BIAS AND RANDOM ERROR

Gordon Guyatt, Roman Jaeschke,
and Maureen O. Meade

IN THIS CHAPTER:

Random Error

Bias

Strategies for Reducing Bias: Therapy and Harm

Our clinical questions have a correct answer that corresponds to an underlying reality or truth. For instance, there is a true underlying magnitude of the impact of β-blockers on mortality in patients with heart failure, of the impact of inhaled steroids on exacerbations in patients with asthma, and of the impact of carotid endarterectomy on incidence of strokes in patients with transient ischemic attacks. Research studies attempt to estimate that underlying truth. Unfortunately, however, we will never know what that true impact really is (Table 5-1). Studies may be flawed in their design or conduct and introduce *systematic error (bias)*. Even if a study could be perfectly designed and executed, we would remain uncertain whether we had arrived at the underlying truth. The next section explains why.

RANDOM ERROR

Consider a perfectly balanced coin. Every time we flip the coin, the *probability* of its landing with head up or tail up is equal—50%. Assume, however, that we as investigators do not know that the coin is perfectly balanced—in fact, we have

TABLE 5-1

Study Results and the Underlying Truth

Result from a completed study yields an apparent treatment effect

- Technical term: point estimate (of the underlying truth)
- Example: relative risk of death is 0.75 or 75%
- Possible underlying truth 1: reduction in relative risk of death really is 25%
- Possible underlying truth 2: reduction in relative risk of death is appreciably less than or greater than 25%

Possible explanations for inaccuracy of the point estimate

- Random error (synonym: chance)
- Systematic error (synonyms: bias, limitation in validity)

no idea how well balanced it is, and we would like to find out. We can state our question formally: What is the true underlying probability of a resulting head or tail on any given coin flip? Our first experiment addressing this question is a series of 10 coin flips; the result: 8 heads and 2 tails. What are we to conclude? Taking our result at face value, we infer that the coin is very unbalanced (that is, biased in such a way that it yields heads more often than tails) and that the probability of heads on any given flip is 80%.

Few would be happy with this conclusion. The reason for our discomfort is that we know that the world is not constructed so that a perfectly balanced coin will always yield 5 heads and 5 tails in any given set of 10 coin flips. Rather, the result is subject to the play of chance, otherwise known as *random error*. Some of the time, 10 flips of a perfectly balanced coin will yield 8 heads. On occasion, 9 of 10 flips will turn up heads. On rare occasions, we will find heads on all 10 flips. Figure 5-1 shows the actual distribution of heads and tails in repeated series of coin flips.

FIGURE 5-1

Theoretical Distribution of Results of an Infinite Number of Repetitions of 10 Flips of an Unbiased Coin

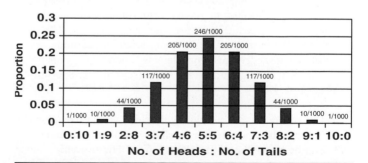

What if the 10 coin flips yield 5 heads and 5 tails? Our awareness of the play of chance leaves us uncertain that the coin is a true one: a series of 10 coin flips of a very biased coin (a true probability of heads of .8, for instance) could, by chance, yield 5 heads and 5 tails.

Let us say that a funding agency, intrigued by the results of our first small experiment, provides us with resources to conduct a larger study. This time, we increase the sample size of our experiment markedly, conducting a series of 1000 coin flips. If we end up with 500 heads and 500 tails, are we ready to conclude that we are dealing with a true coin? Not quite. We know that, were the true underlying probability of heads 51%, we would sometimes see 1000 coin flips yield the result we have just observed.

We can apply the above logic to the results of experiments addressing health care issues in humans. A *randomized controlled trial (RCT)* shows that 10 of 100 treated patients die in the course of treatment, as do 20 of 100 control patients. Does treatment really reduce the death rate by 50%? Maybe, but awareness of chance will leave us with considerable uncertainty about the magnitude of the *treatment effect*—and perhaps about whether treatment helps at all.

To use an actual example, in a study of congestive heart failure, 228 of 1320 (17%) patients with moderate to severe heart failure allocated to receive *placebo* died, as did 156 of 1327 (12%) allocated to receive bisoprolol.[1] Although the true underlying reduction in the *relative risk* of dying is likely to be in the vicinity of the 32% suggested by the study, we must acknowledge that considerable uncertainty remains about the true magnitude of the effect (see Chapter 8, Confidence Intervals).

Let us remember the question with which we started: Why is it that no matter how powerful and well designed our experiment, we will never be sure of the true treatment effect? The answer is: chance.

BIAS

What do we mean when we say that a study is valid or believable? In this book, we use *validity* as a technical term that relates to the magnitude of bias. In contrast to random error, bias leads to systematic deviations (ie, the error has direction) from the underlying truth. In studies of treatment or *harm*, bias leads to either an underestimate or an overestimate of the underlying benefit or harm (Table 5-2).

Bias may intrude as a result of differences, other than the *experimental intervention*, between patients in treatment and *control groups* at the time they enter a study. At the start of a study, each patient, if left untreated, is destined to do well—or poorly. To do poorly means to have an adverse event—say, a stroke—during the course of the study. We often refer to the adverse event that is the focus of a study as the *target outcome* or *target event*. Bias will result if treated and control patients differ in substantive outcome-associated ways at the start of the study. For instance, if control-group patients have more severe atherosclerosis or are older than their counterparts, their destiny will be to have a greater proportion of adverse events than those in the intervention or treatment group,

TABLE 5-2

How Can a Study of an Intervention (Treatment) Be Biased?

Intervention and control groups may be different at the start

Example: patients in control group are sicker or older

Intervention and control groups may, independent of the experimental treatment, become different as the study proceeds

Example: patients in the intervention group receive effective additional medication

Intervention and control groups may differ, independent of treatment, at the end

Example: more sick patients lost to follow-up in the intervention group and the results of the study will be biased in favor of the treatment group; that is, the study will yield a systematically greater estimate of the treatment effect than would be obtained were the study groups alike prognostically.

Even if patients in the intervention and control groups begin the study with the same *prognosis*, the result may still be biased. This will occur if, for instance, effective interventions are differentially administered to treatment and control groups. For instance, in a study of a novel agent for the *prevention* of complications of atherosclerosis, the intervention group might receive more intensive statin therapy than the control group.

Finally, patients may begin prognostically similar, and stay prognostically similar, but the study may end with a biased result. This could occur if the study loses patients to *follow-up* (see Chapter 6, Therapy [Randomized Trials]), or because a study is *stopped early* because of an apparent large treatment effect.

STRATEGIES FOR REDUCING BIAS: THERAPY AND HARM

We have noted that bias arises from differences in *prognostic factors* in treatment and control groups at the start of a study, or from differences in prognosis that arise as a study proceeds. What can investigators do to reduce these biases? Table 5-3 summarizes the available strategies in RCTs of therapy and *observational studies* addressing issues of harm.

When studying new treatments, investigators often have a great deal of control. They can reduce the likelihood of differences in the distribution of prognostic features in treated and untreated patients at baseline by *randomly allocating* patients to the 2 groups. They can markedly reduce placebo effects by administering identical-appearing but biologically inert treatments—placebos—to control-group patients. *Blinding* clinicians to whether patients are receiving active or placebo therapy can eliminate the risk of important *cointerven-*

TABLE 5-3

Ways of Reducing Bias in Studies of Therapy and Harm

Source of Bias	Therapy: Strategy for Reducing Bias	Harm: Strategy for Reducing Bias
Differences Observed at the Start of the Study		
Treatment and control patients differ in prognosis	Randomization	Statistical adjustment for prognostic factors in the analysis of data
	Randomization with stratification	Matching
Differences That Arise as the Study Proceeds		
Placebo effects	Blinding of patients	Choice of outcomes (such as mortality) less subject to placebo effects
Cointervention	Blinding of caregivers	Documentation of treatment differences and statistical adjustment
Bias in assessment of outcome	Blinding of assessors of outcome	Choice of outcomes (such as mortality) less subject to observer bias
Differences at the Completion of the Study		
Loss to follow-up	Ensuring complete follow-up	Ensuring complete follow-up
Stopping study early because of large effect	Completing study as initially planned	
Omitting patients who did not receive assigned treatment	Adhering to intention-to-treat principle and including all patients in the arm to which they are randomized	

tions, and blinding outcome assessors minimizes bias in the assessment of *event rates*.

In general, investigators studying the effect of potentially harmful exposures have far less control than those investigating the effects of potentially beneficial treatments. They must be content to compare patients whose exposure is determined by their choice or circumstances, and they can address potential differences in patients' fate only by statistical adjustment for known prognostic factors. Blinding is impossible, so their best defense against placebo effects and bias in outcome assessment is to choose *endpoints*, such as death, that are less subject to these biases. Investigators addressing both sets of questions can reduce bias by minimizing loss to follow-up (see Table 5-1).

These general rules do not always apply. Sometimes, investigators studying a new treatment find it difficult or impossible to randomize patients to treatment and control groups. Under such circumstances, they choose observational study designs, and clinicians must apply the validity criteria developed for questions of harm to such studies.

Similarly, if the potentially harmful exposure is a drug with beneficial effects, investigators may be able to randomize patients to intervention and control groups. In this case, clinicians can apply the validity criteria designed for therapy questions to the study. Whether for issues of therapy or harm, the strength of inference from RCTs will almost invariably be far greater than the strength of inference from observational studies.

Reference

1. CIBIS-II Investigators and Committees. The Cardiac Insufficiency Bisoprolol Study II (CIBIS-II): a randomised trial. *Lancet*. 1999;353(9146):9-13.

6

THERAPY (RANDOMIZED TRIALS)

Gordon Guyatt, Sharon Straus, Maureen O. Meade,
Regina Kunz, Deborah J. Cook, PJ Devereaux,
and John Ioannidis

IN THIS CHAPTER:

How Can I Apply the Results to Patient Care?

Were the Study Patients Similar to the Patient in My Practice?

Were All Patient-Important Outcomes Considered?

Are the Likely Treatment Benefits Worth the Potential Harm and Costs?

Clinical Resolution

CLINICAL SCENARIO

A Patient With Coronary Disease and a Gastrointestinal Bleed: How Can I Best Help Avoid Vascular Events and Minimize Bleeding Risk?

You are a general internist following a 62-year-old man with peptic ulcer disease and stable angina for whom you have been prescribing low-dose aspirin, a statin, an angiotensin-converting enzyme inhibitor, and as-needed nitrates. Recently, the patient developed an upper gastrointestinal bleed. Biopsy done at endoscopy was negative for *Helicobacter pylori*. In hospital, the gastroenterologist looking after your patient changed the aspirin to clopidogrel (and supported his action by citing a systematic review of thienopyridine derivatives, including clopidogrel, in high-risk vascular patients that found a decrease in the odds of a gastrointestinal bleed compared with aspirin; odds ratio, 0.71; 95% *confidence interval* [*CI*], 0.59-0.86).[1]

You use *ACP Journal Club* to browse the medical literature and, reviewing the patient's story, you recall a recent article that may be relevant. The patient is currently stable and you ask him to return in a week for further review of his medications.

FINDING THE EVIDENCE

Evidence from populations with vascular disease suggests that clopidogrel is likely to be similar, if not superior, to aspirin in its ability to prevent vascular events in patients with stable angina,[2] allowing you to focus on prevention of bleeding. You therefore formulate the relevant question: in a patient with previous aspirin-associated ulcer, is clopidogrel effective in preventing recurrent ulcer bleeding? Searching *ACP Journal Club* in your medical library's Ovid system with the terms "clopidogrel" and "gastrointestinal bleeding" identifies 3 articles, one of which turns out to be your target: "Aspirin plus esomeprazole reduced recurrent ulcer bleeding more than clopidogrel in high-risk patients."[3] You print a copy of this and the original full-text article.[4]

This article describes a *randomized, placebo*-controlled trial including 320 patients with endoscopically confirmed ulcer bleeding, either negative test results for *H pylori* or successful eradication of *H pylori*, and anticipated regular use of antiplatelet therapy. Participants were *randomly allocated* to clopidogrel 75 mg daily and placebo or to aspirin 80 mg and esomeprazole (a potent proton-pump inhibitor) 20 mg twice daily for 12 months. The primary *outcome* was recurrent ulcer bleeding, and secondary outcomes included lower gastrointestinal bleeding and adverse effects.

The Users' Guides

Table 6-1 presents our usual 3-step approach to using an article from the medical literature to guide your practice. You will find these criteria useful for a variety of therapy-related questions, including treating symptomatic illnesses (eg, asthma or arthritis), *preventing* distant complications of illness (eg, cardiovascular death after myocardial infarction), and *screening* for silent but treatable disease (eg, colon cancer screening).

If the answer to one key question (Were patients randomized?) is no, some of the other questions (Was randomization *concealed*? Were patients analyzed in the groups to which they were randomized?) will lose their relevance. As you will see, nonrandomized *observational studies* yield far weaker inferences than *randomized controlled trials* (*RCTs*). Nevertheless, clinicians must use the best evidence available in managing their patients, even if the quality of that evidence is limited (see Chapter 2, The Philosophy of Evidence-Based Medicine). The criteria in Chapter 9 (Harm [Observational Studies]) will help you assess an observational study addressing a potential treatment that has not yet been evaluated in an RCT.

TABLE 6-1

Users' Guides for an Article About Therapy

Are the results valid?

- Did intervention and control groups start with the same prognosis?
  - Were patients randomized?
  - Was randomization concealed?
  - Were patients in the study groups similar with respect to known prognostic factors?
- Was prognostic balance maintained as the study progressed?
  - To what extent was the study blinded?
- Were the groups prognostically balanced at the study's completion?
  - Was follow-up complete?
  - Were patients analyzed in the groups to which they were ran- domized?
  - Was the trial stopped early?

What are the results?

- How large was the treatment effect?
- How precise was the estimate of the treatment effect?

How can I apply the results to patient care?

- Were the study patients similar to my patient?
- Were all patient-important outcomes considered?
- Are the likely treatment benefits worth the potential harm and costs?

ARE THE RESULTS VALID?

Did Intervention and Control Groups Start With the Same Prognosis?

Were Patients Randomized?
Consider the question of whether hospital care prolongs life. A study finds that more sick people die in the hospital than in the community. We would easily reject the naive conclusion

that hospital care kills because we understand that hospitalized patients are sicker than patients in the community.

Although the logic of prognostic balance is vividly clear in comparing hospitalized patients with those in the community, it may be less obvious in other contexts. Until recently, clinicians and epidemiologists (and almost everyone else) believed that hormone replacement therapy (HRT) could decrease the *risk* of coronary events (death and myocardial infarction) in postmenopausal women. The belief arose from the results of many studies that found women taking HRT to have a decreased risk of coronary events.[5] Results of the first large randomized trial of women with established coronary artery disease (CAD) provided a surprise: HRT failed to reduce the risk of coronary events.[6] Even more recently, the Women's Health Initiative demonstrated that HRT also failed in the primary prevention of CAD.[7]

Other surprises generated by randomized trials include the demonstration that antioxidant vitamins fail to reduce gastrointestinal cancer[8]—and one such agent, vitamin E, may actually increase all-cause mortality[9]—and that a variety of initially promising drugs increase mortality in patients with heart failure.[10-15] Such surprises occur periodically when investigators conduct randomized trials to test the observations from studies in which patients and physicians determine which treatment a patient receives.[16]

The reason that studies in which patient or physician preference determines whether a patient receives treatment or control (observational studies) often yield misleading results is that morbidity and mortality result from many causes, of which treatment is only one. Treatment studies attempt to determine the impact of an intervention on such events as stroke, myocardial infarction, and death—occurrences that we call the trial's *target outcomes*. A patient's age, the underlying severity of illness, the presence of *comorbidity*, and a host of other factors typically determine the frequency with which a trial's target outcome occurs (*prognostic factors* or *determinants of outcome*). If prognostic factors—either those we know about or those we do not know about—prove unbalanced between a trial's treatment and *control groups*, the study's outcome will be biased, either underestimating or overestimating the treatment's effect. Because known prognostic factors often influence clinicians' recommendations and patients' decisions about taking treatment, observational studies often yield biased results.

Observational studies can theoretically match patients, either in the selection of patients for study or in the subsequent statistical analysis, for known prognostic factors (see Chapter 9, Harm [Obervational Studies], and Chapter 5, Why Study Results Mislead: Bias and Random Error). The power of randomization is that treatment and control groups are more likely to be balanced with respect to both known and unknown determinants of outcome.

> What was the cause of *bias* in the HRT observational studies? Evidence suggests that women who took HRT enjoyed a higher socioeconomic status.[17] Their apparent benefit from HRT was probably due to factors such as a healthier lifestyle and a greater sense of control over life. Whatever the explanation, we are now confident that it was their previous *prognosis*, rather than the HRT, that led to lower rates of CAD.

Although randomization is a powerful technique, it does not always succeed in creating groups with similar prognosis. Investigators may make mistakes that compromise randomization, or randomization may fail because of simple bad luck. The next 2 sections address these issues.

Was Randomization Concealed?

Some years ago, a group of Australian investigators undertook a randomized trial of open vs laparoscopic appendectomy.[18] The trial ran smoothly during the day. At night, however, the attending surgeon's presence was required for the laparoscopic procedure but not the open one, and limited operating room availability made the longer laparoscopic procedure an annoyance. Reluctant to call in a consultant, the residents sometimes adopted what they saw as a practical solution. When an eligible patient appeared, the residents held the semiopaque envelopes containing the study assignment up to the light. They opened the first envelope that dictated an open procedure. The first eligible patient in the morning would then be allocated to the laparoscopic appendectomy group according to the passed-over envelope (D. Wall, written communication, June 2000). If patients who presented at night were sicker than those who presented during the day, the residents' behavior would bias the results against the open procedure.

When those enrolling patients are unaware and cannot control the arm to which the patient is allocated, we refer to randomization as concealed. In unconcealed trials, those responsible for recruitment may systematically enroll sicker—or less sick—patients to either treatment or control groups. This behavior will defeat the purpose of randomization and the study will yield a biased result.[19-21] Careful investigators will ensure that randomization is concealed through strategies such as remote randomization, in which the individual recruiting the patient makes a call to a methods center to discover the arm of the study to which the patient is assigned.

Were Patients in the Treatment and Control Groups Similar With Respect to Known Prognostic Factors?

The purpose of randomization is to create groups whose prognosis, with respect to the target outcomes, is similar. Sometimes, through bad luck, randomization will fail to achieve this goal. The smaller the sample size, the more likely the trial will have prognostic imbalance.

Picture a trial testing a new treatment for heart failure enrolling patients in New York Heart Association functional class III and class IV. Patients in class IV have a much worse prognosis than those in class III. The trial is small, with only 8 patients. One would not be surprised if all 4 class III patients were allocated to the treatment group and all 4 class IV patients were allocated to the control group. Such a result of the allocation process would seriously bias the study in favor of the treatment. Were the trial to enroll 800 patients, one would be startled if randomization placed all 400 class III patients in the treatment arm. The larger the sample size, the more likely randomization will achieve its goal of prognostic balance.

You can check how effectively randomization has balanced prognostic factors by looking for a display of patient characteristics of the treatment and control groups at the study's commencement—the baseline or entry prognostic features. Although we will never know whether similarity exists for the unknown prognostic factors, we are reassured when the known prognostic factors are well balanced.

All is not lost if the treatment groups are not similar at baseline. Statistical techniques permit adjustment of the study result for baseline differences. *Adjusted analyses* may not be preferable to unadjusted analyses, but when both analyses generate the same conclusion, readers gain confidence in the *validity* of the study result.

Was Prognostic Balance Maintained as the Study Progressed?
To What Extent Was the Study Blinded?

If randomization succeeds, treatment and control groups in a study begin with a similar prognosis. Randomization, however, provides no guarantees that the 2 groups will remain prognostically balanced. *Blinding* is, if possible, the optimal strategy for maintaining prognostic balance.

Table 6-2 describes 5 groups involved in clinical trials that, ideally, will remain unaware of whether patients are receiving the *experimental therapy* or control therapy. You are probably aware that patients who take a treatment that they believe is effective may feel and perform better than those who do not, even if the treatment has no biologic activity. Although the magnitude and consistency of this *placebo effect* remain uncertain,[22-25] investigators interested in determining the biologic impact of a pharmacologic or nonpharmacologic treatment will ensure patients are blind to treatment allocation. Similarly, rigorous research designs will ensure blinding of those collecting, evaluating, and analyz-

TABLE 6-2

Five Groups That Should, if Possible, Be Blind to Treatment Assignment

Patients	To avoid placebo effects
Clinicians	To prevent differential administration of therapies that affect the outcome of interest (cointervention)
Data collectors	To prevent bias in data collection
Adjudicators of outcome	To prevent bias in decisions about whether or not a patient has had an outcome of interest
Data analysts	To avoid bias in decisions regarding data analysis

ing data (Table 6-2). Demonstrations of bias introduced by unblinding—such as the results of a trial in multiple sclerosis in which a treatment benefit judged by unblinded outcome assessors disappeared when adjudicators of outcome were blinded[26]—highlight the importance of blinding. The more that judgment is involved in determining whether a patient has had a target outcome (blinding is less crucial in studies in which the outcome is all-cause mortality, for instance), the more important blinding becomes.

Finally, differences in patient care other than the intervention under study—*cointervention*—can, if they affect study outcomes, bias the results. Effective blinding eliminates the possibility of either conscious or unconscious differential administration of effective interventions to treatment and control groups. When effective blinding is not possible, documentation of potential cointervention becomes important.

Were the Groups Prognostically Balanced at the Study's Completion?

Unfortunately, investigators can ensure concealed random allocation and effective blinding and still fail to achieve an unbiased result.

Was Follow-up Complete?

Ideally, at the conclusion of a trial, you will know the status of each patient with respect to the target outcome. The greater the number of patients whose outcome is unknown—patients lost to follow-up—the more a study's validity is potentially compromised. The reason is that patients who are lost often have different prognoses from those who are retained—they may disappear because they have adverse outcomes or because they are doing well and so did not return for assessment.[27]

When does loss to follow-up seriously threaten validity? Rules of thumb (you may run across thresholds such as 20%) are misleading. Consider 2 hypothetical randomized trials, each of which enters 1000 patients into both treatment and control groups, of whom 30 (3%) are lost to follow-up (Table 6-3). In

TABLE 6-3

When Does Loss to Follow-up Seriously Threaten Validity?

	Trial A		Trial B	
	Treatment	**Control**	**Treatment**	**Control**
Number of patients randomized	1000	1000	1000	1000
Number (%) lost to follow-up	30 (3)	30 (3)	30 (3)	30 (3)
Number (%) of deaths	200 (20)	400 (40)	30 (3)	60 (6)
RRR not counting patients lost to follow-up	0.2/0.4 = 0.50		0.03/0.06 = 0.50	
RRR—worst-case scenario[a]	0.17/0.4 = 0.43		0.00/0.06 = 0	

Abbreviation: RRR, relative risk reduction.

[a]The worst-case scenario assumes that all patients allocated to the treatment group and lost to follow-up died and all patients allocated to the control group and lost to follow-up survived.

trial A, treated patients die at half the rate of the control group (200 vs 400), a *relative risk reduction (RRR)* of 50%. To what extent does the loss to follow-up potentially threaten our inference that treatment reduces the death rate by half? If we assume the worst (ie, that all treated patients lost to follow-up died), the number of deaths in the experimental group would be 230 (23%). If there were no deaths among the control patients who were lost to follow-up, our best estimate of the effect of treatment in reducing the risk of death drops from 200/400, or 50%, to (400 − 230)/400 or 170/400, or 43%. Thus, even assuming the worst makes little difference to the best estimate of the magnitude of the *treatment effect*. Our inference is therefore secure.

Contrast this with trial B. Here, the reduction in the *relative risk (RR)* of death is also 50%. In this case, however, the total number of deaths is much lower; of the treated patients, 30 die, and the number of deaths in control patients is 60. In trial B, if we make the same worst-case assumption about the fate of the patients lost to follow-up, the results would change markedly. If we assume that all patients initially allocated to treatment—but subsequently lost to follow-up—die, the number of deaths among treated patients rises from 30 to 60, which is exactly equal to the number of control group deaths. Let us assume that this assumption is accurate. Because we would have 60 deaths in both treatment and control groups, the effect of treatment drops to 0. Because of this dramatic change in the treatment effect (50% RRR if we ignore those lost to follow-up; 0% RRR if we assume all patients in the treatment group who were lost to follow-up died), the 3% loss to follow-up in trial B threatens our inference about the magnitude of the RRR.

Of course, this worst-case scenario is unlikely. When a worst-case scenario, were it true, substantially alters the results, you must judge the plausibility of a markedly different outcome *event rate* in the treatment and control group patients lost to follow-up.

In conclusion, loss to follow-up potentially threatens a study's validity. If assuming a worst-case scenario does not change the inferences arising from study results, then loss to follow-up is not a problem. If such an assumption would significantly alter the results, the extent to which validity is compromised depends on how likely it is that treatment patients lost to follow-up did badly while control patients lost to follow-up did well. That decision is a matter of judgment.

Was the Trial Stopped Early?

Although it is becoming increasingly popular, stopping trials early when one sees an apparent large benefit is risky.[28] Trials terminated early will compromise randomization if they stop at a "random high" when prognostic factors temporarily favor the intervention group. Particularly when sample size and the number of events are small, trials stopped early run the risk of greatly overestimating the treatment effect.[29]

Were Patients Analyzed in the Groups to Which They Were Randomized?

Investigators can also undermine randomization if they omit from the analysis patients who do not receive their assigned treatment or, worse yet, count events that occur in *nonadherent* patients who were assigned to treatment against the control group. Such analyses will bias the results if the reasons for nonadherence are related to prognosis. In a number of randomized trials, patients who did not adhere to their assigned drug regimens have fared worse than those who took their medication as instructed, even after taking into account all known prognostic factors and even when their medications were placebos.[30-35] When adherent patients are destined to have a better outcome, omitting those who do not receive assigned treatment undermines the unbiased comparison provided by randomization. Investigators prevent this bias when they follow the *intention-to-treat* principle and analyze all patients in the group to which they were randomized.[36]

USING THE GUIDE

Returning to our opening clinical scenario, did the experimental and control groups begin the study with a similar prognosis? The study was randomized and allocation was concealed; 320 patients participated and 99% were followed up. The investigators followed the intention-to-treat principle, including all patients in the arm to which they were randomized, and stopped when they reached the planned sample size. There were more patients who smoked (13% vs 8.2%) and regularly consumed alcohol (8.1% vs 5%) in the clopidogrel group compared with the aspirin-esomeprazole group. This could bias the results in favor of the aspirin-esomeprazole, and the investigators do not provide an adjusted analysis for the baseline differences. Clinicians, patients, data collectors, outcomes assessors, and data analysts were all blind to allocation.

The final assessment of validity is never a yes-or-no decision. Rather, think of validity as a continuum ranging from strong studies that are very likely to yield an accurate estimate of the treatment effect to weak studies that are very likely to yield a biased estimate of effect. Inevitably, the judgment as to where a study lies in this continuum involves some subjectivity. In this case, despite uncertainty about baseline differences between the groups, we conclude that the methods were strong.

What Are the Results?

How Large Was the Treatment Effect?

Most frequently, RCTs carefully monitor how often patients experience some adverse event or outcome. Examples of these dichotomous outcomes (yes-or-no outcomes, ones that either happen or do not happen) include cancer recurrence, myocardial infarction, and death. Patients either have an event or they do not, and the article reports the proportion of patients who develop such events. Consider, for example, a study in which 20% of a control group died, but only 15% of those receiving a new treatment died (Table 6-4). How might one express these results?

One possibility would be the absolute difference (known as the *absolute risk reduction [ARR]*, or *risk difference*), between the proportion who died in the control group (*baseline risk* or *control group risk [CGR]*) and the proportion who died in the experimental group (*experimental group risk [EGR]*), or CGR – EGR = 0.20 – 0.15 = 0.05. Another way to express the impact of treatment is as an RR: the risk of events among patients receiving the new treatment relative to that risk among patients in the control group, or EGR/CGR = 0.15/0.20 = 0.75.

The most commonly reported measure of dichotomous treatment effects is the complement of the RR, the RRR. It is expressed as a percentage: 1 – (EGR/CGR) × 100% = (1 – 0.75) × 100% = 25%. An

TABLE 6-4

Results From a Hypothetical Randomized Trial

	Outcome		
Exposure	Death	Survival	Total
Treatment (experimental)	15	85	100
Control	20	80	100

Control group risk (CGR): 20/100 = 20%.

Experimental group risk (EGR): 15/100 = 15%.

Absolute risk reduction or risk difference: CGR – EGR, 20% – 15% = 5%.

Relative risk: EGR/CGR = (15/100)/(20/100) × 100% = 75%.

Relative risk reduction: [1 – (EGR/CGR)] × 100% = 1 – 75% = 25%.

RRR of 25% means that the new treatment reduced the risk of death by 25% relative to that occurring among control patients; the greater the RRR, the more effective the therapy. Investigators may compute the RR over a period of time, as in a *survival analysis*, and call it a *hazard ratio* (see Chapter 7, Does Treatment Lower Risk? Understanding the Results). When people do not specify whether they are talking about RRR or ARR—for instance, "Drug X was 30% effective in reducing the risk of death," or "The efficacy of the vaccine was 92%"—they are almost invariably talking about RRR (see Chapter 7, Does Treatment Lower Risk? Understanding the Results, for more detail about how the RRR results in a subjective impression of a larger treatment effect than do other ways of expressing treatment effects).

How Precise Was the Estimate of the Treatment Effect?

We can never be sure of the true risk reduction; the best estimate of the true treatment effect is what we observe in a well-designed randomized trial. This estimate is called a *point estimate* to remind us that, although the true value lies somewhere in its neighborhood, it is unlikely to be precisely correct. Investigators often tell us the neighborhood within which the true effect likely lies by calculating CIs, a range of values within which one can be confident the true effect lies.[37]

We usually use the 95% CI (see Chapter 8, Confidence Intervals). You can consider the 95% CI as defining the range that—assuming the study was well conducted and has minimal bias—includes the true RRR 95% of the time. The true RRR will generally lie beyond these extremes only 5% of the time, a property of the CI that relates closely to the conventional level of *statistical significance* of $P < .05$. We illustrate the use of CIs in the following examples.

Example 1

If a trial randomized 100 patients each to experimental and control groups, and there were 20 deaths in the control group and 15 deaths in the experimental group, the authors would calculate a point estimate for the RRR of 25% [CGR = 20/100 or 0.20, EGR = 15/100 or 0.15, and $1 - EGR/CGR = (1 - 0.75) \times 100 = 25\%$].

You might guess, however, that the true RRR might be much smaller or much greater than 25%, based on a difference of only 5 deaths. In fact, you might surmise that the treatment might provide no benefit (an RRR of 0%) or might even do harm (a negative RRR). And you would be right; in fact, these results are consistent with both an RRR of −38% (that is, patients given the new treatment might be 38% more likely to die than control patients) and an RRR of nearly 59% (that is, patients subsequently receiving the new treatment might have a risk of dying almost 60% less than those who are not treated). In other words, the 95% CI on this RRR is −38% to 59%, and the trial really has not helped us decide whether or not to offer the new treatment.

Example 2

What if the trial enrolled 1000 patients per group rather than 100 patients per group, and the same event rates were observed as before, so that there were 200 deaths in the control group (CGR = 200/1000 = 0.20) and 150 deaths in the experimental group (EGR = 150/1000 = 0.15)? Again, the point estimate of the RRR is 25% (1 − EGR/CGR = 1 − (0.15/0.20) × 100 = 25%).

In this larger trial, you might think that our confidence that the true reduction in risk is close to 25% is much greater, and, again, you would be right. The 95% CI on the RRR for this set of results is all on the positive side of zero and runs from 9% to 41%.

What these examples show is that the larger the sample size of a trial, the larger the number of outcome events and the greater our confidence that the true RRR (or any other measure of effect) is close to what we have observed. In the second example, the lowest plausible value for the RRR was 9% and the highest value was 41%. The point estimate—in this case, 25%—is the one value most likely to represent the true RRR. As one considers values farther and farther from the point estimate, they become less and less consistent with the observed RRR. By the time one crosses the upper or lower boundaries of the 95% CI, the values are very unlikely to represent the true RRR, given the point estimate (that is, the observed RRR). All this, of course, assumes the study has satisfied the validity criteria we discussed earlier.

Figure 6-1 represents the CIs around the point estimate of an RRR of 25% in these 2 examples, with a risk reduction of 0 representing no treatment effect. In both scenarios, the point estimate of the RRR is 25%, but the CI is far narrower in the second scenario.

Not all randomized trials have dichotomous outcomes, nor should they. In a study of respiratory muscle training for patients with chronic airflow limitation, one primary outcome measured how far patients could walk in 6 minutes in an enclosed corridor.[38] This 6-minute walk improved from an average of 406 to 416 m (up 10 m) in the experimental group receiving respiratory muscle training and from 409 to 429 m (up 20 m) in the control

FIGURE 6-1

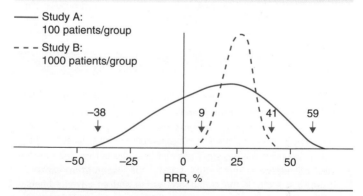

Confidence Intervals in Trials of Various Sample Size

—— Study A:
100 patients/group

- - - Study B:
1000 patients/group

Abbreviations: CI, confidence interval; RRR, relative risk reduction.

Two studies with the same point estimate, a 25% RRR, but different sample sizes and correspondingly different CIs. The x-axis represents the different possible RRR, and the y-axis represents the likelihood of the true RRR having that particular value. The solid line represents the CI around the first example, in which there were 100 patients per group, and the number of events in active and control was 15 and 20, respectively. The broken line represents the CI around the second example in which there were 1000 patients per group, and the number of events in active and control was 150 and 200, respectively.

group. The point estimate for improvement in the 6-minute walk due to respiratory muscle training therefore was negative, at −10 m (or a 10-m difference in favor of the control group).

Here, too, you should look for the 95% CIs around this difference in changes in exercise capacity and consider their implications. The investigators tell us that the lower boundary of the 95% CI was −26 (that is, the results are consistent with a difference of 26 m in favor of the control treatment) and the upper boundary was +5 m. Even in the best of circumstances, patients are unlikely to perceive adding 5 m to the 400 recorded at the start of the trial as important, and this result effectively excludes an important benefit of respiratory muscle training as applied in this study.

It will not surprise you that the larger the sample size, the narrower the CI. If you want to learn more about CIs, including finding out when the sample size is sufficiently large, see Chapter 8, Confidence Intervals.

Having determined the magnitude and precision of the treatment effect, clinicians can turn to the final question of how to apply the article's results to their patients.

USING THE GUIDE

Using the raw numbers provided in the article, 1 of 159 people (0.6%) in the aspirin-esomeprazole group and 13 of the 161 people (8%) in the clopidogrel group experienced a recurrence of ulcer. The RRR is 92%, and the 95% CI extends from 41% to 99%. The very large effect and the small number of events somewhat reduce your confidence in this result; 4.4% of the aspirin-esomeprazole group and 9.4% of the clopidogrel group had an adverse effect (defined as dyspepsia or an allergy). The investigators also reported that 11 patients in the aspirin-esomeprazole group and 9 patients in the clopidogrel group experienced recurrent ischemic events.

HOW CAN I APPLY THE RESULTS TO PATIENT CARE?

Were the Study Patients Similar to the Patient in My Practice?

Often, the patient before you has different attributes or characteristics from those enrolled in the trial. He or she may be older or younger, sicker or less sick, or may have comorbid disease that would have excluded him or her from participation in the research study. If the patient qualified for enrollment in the study, you can apply the results with considerable confidence.

What if that individual does not meet a study's eligibility criteria? The study result probably applies even if, for example, he or she was 2 years too old for the study, had more severe disease, had previously been treated with a competing therapy, or had a comorbid condition. A better approach than rigidly applying the study's *inclusion and exclusion criteria* is to ask whether there is some compelling reason why the results do not apply to the patient. You usually will not find a compelling reason, and most often you can generalize the results to your patient with confidence.

A related issue has to do with the extent to which we can generalize findings from a study using a particular drug to another closely (or not so closely) related agent. The issue of drug class effects and how conservative one should be in assuming class effects remains controversial. Generalizing findings of surgical treatment may be even riskier. Randomized trials of carotid endarterectomy, for instance, demonstrate much lower perioperative rates of stroke and death than one might expect in one's own community.[39]

A final issue arises when a patient fits the features of a subgroup of patients in the trial report. We encourage you to be skeptical of *subgroup analyses*.[40] The treatment is likely to benefit the subgroup more or less than the other patients only if the difference in the effects of treatment in the subgroups is large and very unlikely to occur by chance. Even when these conditions apply, the results may be misleading if investigators did not specify their hypotheses before the study began, if they had a very large number of hypotheses, or if other studies fail to replicate the finding.

Were All Patient-Important Outcomes Considered?

Treatments are indicated when they provide important benefits. Demonstrating that a bronchodilator produces small increments in forced expired volume in patients with chronic airflow limitation, that a vasodilator improves cardiac output in heart failure patients, or that a lipid-lowering agent improves lipid profiles does not provide a sufficient reason for administering these drugs. Here, investigators have chosen *substitute* or *surrogate outcomes* rather than those that patients would consider important. What clinicians and patients require is evidence that the treatments improve outcomes that are important to patients (*patient-important outcomes*), such as reducing shortness of breath during the activities required for daily living, avoiding hospitalization for heart failure, or decreasing the risk of myocardial infarction.[41]

Trials of the impact of antiarrhythmic drugs after myocardial infarction illustrate the danger of using *substitute outcomes* or *endpoints*. Because such drugs had demonstrated a reduction in abnormal ventricular depolarizations (the substitute endpoints), it made sense that they should reduce the occurrence of life-threatening arrhythmias. A group of investigators performed randomized trials on 3 agents (encainide, flecainide, and moricizine) that were previously shown to be effective in suppressing the substitute endpoint of abnormal ventricular depolarizations. The investigators had to stop the trials when they discovered that mortality was substantially higher in patients receiving antiarrhythmic treatment than in those receiving placebo.[42,43] Clinicians relying on the substitute endpoint of arrhythmia suppression would have continued to administer the 3 drugs, to the considerable detriment of their patients.

Even when investigators report favorable effects of treatment on one patient-important outcome, you must consider whether there may be deleterious effects on other outcomes. For instance, cancer chemotherapy may lengthen life but decrease its quality. Randomized trials often fail to adequately document the toxicity or adverse effects of the experimental intervention.[44]

Composite endpoints represent a final dangerous trend in presenting outcomes. Like surrogate outcomes, composite endpoints are attractive for reducing sample size and decreasing length of follow-up. Unfortunately, they can mislead. We may find that a trial that reduced a composite outcome of death, renal failure requiring dialysis, and doubling of serum creatinine level actually demonstrated a trend toward increased mortality with the experimental therapy and showed convincing effects only on doubling of serum creatinine level.[45]

Another long-neglected outcome is the resource implications of alternative management strategies. Health care systems face increasing resource constraints that mandate careful attention to *economic analysis.*

Are the Likely Treatment Benefits Worth the Potential Harm and Costs?

If you can apply the study's results to a patient, and its outcomes are important, the next question concerns whether the probable treatment benefits are worth the effort that you and the patient must put into the enterprise. A 25% reduction in the RR of death may sound quite impressive, but its impact on your patient and practice may nevertheless be minimal. This notion is illustrated by using a concept called *number needed to treat (NNT)*, the number of patients who must receive an intervention of therapy during a specific period to prevent 1 adverse outcome or produce 1 positive outcome.[46]

The impact of a treatment is related not only to its RRR but also to the risk of the adverse outcome it is designed to prevent. One large trial in myocardial infarction suggests that tissue plasminogen activator (tPA) administration reduces the RR of death by approximately 12% in comparison to streptokinase.[47] Table 6-5 considers 2 patients presenting with acute myocardial infarction associated with elevation of ST segments on their electrocardiograms.

In the first case, a 40-year-old man presents with electrocardiographic findings suggesting an inferior myocardial

TABLE 6-5

Considerations in the Decision to Treat 2 Patients With Myocardial Infarction With tPA or Streptokinase

	Risk of Death 1 Year After MI With Streptokinase (CER)	Risk With tPA (EGR) (ARR = CGR – EGR)	Number Needed to Treat (100/ARR When ARR is Expressed as a Percentage)
40-Year-old man with small MI	2%	1.76% (0.24% or 0.0024)	417
70-Year-old man with large MI and heart failure	40%	35.2% (4.8% or 0.048)	21

Abbreviations: ARR, absolute risk reduction; CGR, control group risk; EGR, experimental group risk; tPA, tissue plasminogen activator; MI, myocardial infarction.

infarction. You find no signs of heart failure, and the patient is in normal sinus rhythm, with a rate of 90/min. This individual's risk of death in the first year after infarction may be as low as 2%. In comparison to streptokinase, tPA would reduce this risk by 12% to 1.76%, an ARR of 0.24% (0.0024). The inverse of this ARR (that is, 100 divided by the ARR expressed as a percentage) is equal to the number of such patients we would have to treat to prevent 1 event (in this case, to prevent 1 death after a mild heart attack in a low-risk patient), the NNT. In this case, we would have to treat approximately 417 such patients to save a single life (100/0.24 = 417). Given the small increased risk of intracerebral hemorrhage associated with tPA, and its additional cost, many clinicians might prefer streptokinase in this patient.

In the second case, a 70-year-old man presents with electrocardiographic signs of anterior myocardial infarction with pulmonary edema. His risk of dying in the subsequent year is approximately 40%. A 12% RRR of death in such a high-risk patient generates an ARR of 4.8% (0.048), and we would have to treat only 21 such individuals to avert a premature death (100/4.8 = 20.8). Many clinicians would consider tPA the preferable agent for this man.

A key element of the decision to start therapy, therefore, is to consider the patient's risk of the adverse event if left untreated.

For any given RRR, the higher the probability that a patient will experience an adverse outcome if we do not treat, the more likely the patient will benefit from treatment and the fewer such patients we need to treat to prevent 1 adverse outcome (see Chapter 7, Does Treatment Lower Risk? Understanding the Results). Knowing the NNT helps clinicians in the process of weighing the benefits and downsides associated with the management options.

Tradeoff of benefit and risk also requires an accurate assessment of treatment adverse effects. Randomized trials, with relatively small sample sizes, are unsuitable for detecting rare but catastrophic adverse effects of therapy. Clinicians must often look to other sources of information—often characterized by weaker methodology—to obtain an estimate of the adverse effects of therapy (see Chapter 9, Harm [Observational Studies]).

The *preferences* or *values* that determine the correct choice when weighing benefit and risk are those of the individual patient. Great uncertainty about how best to communicate information to patients and how to incorporate their values into clinical decision making remains. Vigorous investigation of this frontier of evidence-based medicine is, however, under way.

Clinicians may find it tempting to turn to the article's authors for guidance about tradeoffs between benefits and risks. Because of the possibility of conflict of interest, this can be dangerous. Prudence will dictate arriving at your own evaluation, often after consulting a reliable source free of conflicts (see Chapter 4, Finding the Evidence).

CLINICAL RESOLUTION

The study that we identified showed a decrease in the recurrence of ulcer bleeding in high-risk patients receiving aspirin-esomeprazole in comparison with those taking clopidogrel. The authors also found that more people in the clopidogrel group experienced an adverse effect from the therapy and that there was no significant difference in the risk of ischemic events, although the small number of outcomes leaves any inferences from this result extremely weak.

Our patient is at a high risk of a recurrent ulcer, given his recent gastrointestinal bleed secondary to an aspirin-induced ulcer. His case is similar to those of patients included in this study. You translate the reduction in risk of bleeding into an NNT of approximately 13 (clopidogrel risk of 8.1% – aspirin/esomeprazole of 0.6% = 7.5%; NNT = 100/7.5). Given the very large effect, the NNT using the more conservative boundary of the CI of an RRR of approximately 40—and thus an NNT of approximately 30—may be more realistic. In combination with the reduction in less-important adverse effects, this seems to be a clear patient-important benefit.

The patient found his bleeding episode terrifying, and he also believes that lowering his risk of bleeding by even as little as 3% during a year would be worthwhile. He gulps, however, when you tell him that esomeprazole costs $2.20 per pill, and if he takes the drug as administered in the trial, it will cost him more than $1600 in the next year. You then explain that the investigators' choice of medication leaves some doubt about the best drug to use along with aspirin. Esomeprazole is still under patent, explaining the high cost. The investigators could have chosen omeprazole, a proton-pump inhibitor with marginal differences in effectiveness relative to esomeprazole, which the patient can purchase for approximately half the price. Ultimately, the patient chooses the aspirin/omeprazole combination.

References

1. Hankey G, Sudlow C, Dunbabin D. Thienopyridine derivatives (ticlopidine, clopidogrel) versus aspirin for preventing stroke and other serious vascular events in high vascular risk patients. *Cochrane Database Syst Rev.* 2000;3(1):CD001246.

2. CAPRIE Steering Committee. A randomised, blinded, trial of clopidogrel versus aspirin in patients at risk of ischaemic events (CAPRIE). *Lancet.* 1996;348(9038):1329-1339.

3. Chan K, Peterson W. Aspirin plus esomeprazole reduced recurrent ulcer bleeding more than clopidogrel in high-risk patients. *ACP J Club.* 2005; 143(1):9.

4. Chan K, Ching J, Hung L, et al. Clopidogrel versus aspirin and esomeprazole to prevent recurrent ulcer bleeding. *N Engl J Med.* 2005;352(3):238-244.

5. Stampfer M, Colditz G. Estrogen replacement therapy and coronary heart disease: a quantitative assessment of the epidemiologic evidence. *Prev Med.* 1991;20(1):47-63.

6. Hulley S, Grady D, Bush T, et al. Randomized trial of estrogen plus progestin for secondary prevention of coronary heart disease in postmenopausal women. *JAMA.* 1998;280(7):605-613.

7. Rossouw J, Anderson G, Prentice R, et al. Risks and benefits of estrogen and progestin in healthy menopausal women: principal results from the Women's Health Initiative randomized controlled trial. *JAMA.* 2002; 288(3): 321-323.

8. Vasotec tablets: enalapril maleate. In: *Physician's Desk Reference.* 52nd ed. Montvale, NJ: Medical Economics; 1998:1771-1774.

9. Pitt B, Zannad F, Remme W, et al. The effect of spironolactone on morbidity and mortality in patients with severe heart failure. *N Engl J Med.* 1999;341(10):709-717.

10. The Xamoterol in Severe Heart Failure Group. Xamoterol in severe heart failure. *Lancet.* 1990;336(8706):1-6.

11. Packer M, Carver J, Rodeheffer R, et al. Effects of oral milrinone on mortality in severe chronic heart failure for the PROMISE Study Research Group. *N Engl J Med.* 1991;325(21):1468-1475.

12. Packer M, Rouleau J, Svedberg K, Pitt B, Fisher L. Effect of flosequinan on survival in chronic heart failure: preliminary results of the PROFILE study: the Profile Investigators [abstract]. *Circulation.* 1993;88(suppl 1):I-301.

13. Hampton J, van Veldhuisen D, Kleber F, et al. Randomised study of effect of ibopamine on survival in patients with advanced severe heart failure for the Second Prospective Randomized Study of Ibopamine on Mortality and Efficacy (PRIME II) Investigators. *Lancet.* 1997;349(9057):971-977.

14. Califf R, Adams K, McKenna W, et al. A randomized controlled trial of epoprostenol therapy for severe congestive heart failure: the Flolan International Randomized Survival Trial (FIRST). *Am Heart J.* 1997;134(1):44-54.

15. Haynes R, Mukherjee J, Sackett D, et al. Functional status changes following medical or surgical treatment for cerebral ischemia: results in the EC/IC Bypass Study. *JAMA*. 1987;257(15):2043-2046.

16. Lacchetti C, Ioannidis J, Guyatt G. Surprising results of randomized trials. Chapter 9.2. In: Guyatt G, Rennie D, eds. *Users' Guides to the Medical Literature: A Manual for Evidence-Based Clinical Practice*, 2nd ed. New York, NY: McGraw-Hill, 2008;113-151.

17. Humphrey L, Chan B, Sox H. Postmenopausal hormone replacement therapy and the primary prevention of cardiovascular disease. *Ann Intern Med*. 2002;137(4):273-284.

18. Hansen J, Smithers B, Sachache D, Wall D, Miller B, Menzies B. Laparoscopic versus open appendectomy: prospective randomized trial. *World J Surg*. 1996;20(1):17-20.

19. Schulz K, Chalmers I, Hayes R, Altman D. Empirical evidence of bias: dimensions of methodological quality associated with estimates of treatment effects in controlled trials. *JAMA*. 1995;273(5):408-412.

20. Moher D, Jones A, Cook D, et al. Does quality of reports of randomised trials affect estimates of intervention efficacy reported in meta-analyses? *Lancet*. 1998;352(9128):609-613.

21. Balk EM, Bonis PA, Moskowitz H, et al. Correlation of quality measures with estimates of treatment effect in meta-analyses of randomized controlled trials. *JAMA*. 2002;287(22):2973-2982.

22. Kaptchuk T. Powerful placebo: the dark side of the randomised controlled trial. *Lancet*. 1998;351(9117):1722-1725.

23. Hrobjartsson A, Gotzsche P. Is the placebo powerless? an analysis of clinical trials comparing placebo with no treatment. *N Engl J Med*. 2001;344(21):1594-1602.

24. McRae C, Cherin E, Yamazaki T, et al. Effects of perceived treatment on quality of life and medical outcomes in a double-blind placebo surgery trial. *Arch Gen Psychiatry*. 2004;61(4):412-420.

25. Rana J, Mannam A, Donnell-Fink L, Gervino E, Sellke F, Laham R. Longevity of the placebo effect in the therapeutic angiogenesis and laser myocardial revascularization trials in patients with coronary heart disease. *Am J Cardiol*. 2005;95(12):1456-1459.

26. Noseworthy JH, Ebers GC, Vandervoort MK, Farquhar RE, Yetisir E, Roberts R. The impact of blinding on the results of a randomized, placebo-controlled multiple sclerosis clinical trial. *Neurology*. 1994;44(1):16-20.

27. Ioannidis JP, Bassett R, Hughes MD, Volberding PA, Sacks HS, Lau J. Predictors and impact of patients lost to follow-up in a long-term randomized trial of immediate versus deferred antiretroviral treatment. *J Acquir Immune Defic Syndr Hum Retrovirol*. 1997;16(1):22-30.

28. Montori VM, Devereaux PJ, Adhikari NK, et al. Randomized trials stopped early for benefit: a systematic review. *JAMA*. 2005;294(17):2203-2209.

29. Montori VM, Devereaux PJ, Adhikari NKJ, et al. Randomized trials stopped early for benefit: a systematic review. *JAMA*. 2005;294(17):2203-2209.

30. Coronary Drug Project Research Group. Influence of adherence to treatment and response of cholesterol on mortality in the Coronary Drug Project. *N Engl J Med*. 1980;303(18):1038-1041.

31. Asher W, Harper H. Effect of human chorionic gonadotropin on weight loss, hunger, and feeling of well-being. *Am J Clin Nutr*. 1973;26(2):211-218.

32. Hogarty G, Goldberg S. Drug and sociotherapy in the aftercare of schizophrenic patients: one-year relapse rates. *Arch Gen Psychiatry*. 1973;28(1):54-64.

33. Fuller R, Roth H, Long S. Compliance with disulfiram treatment of alcoholism. *J Chronic Dis*. 1983;36(2):161-170.

34. Pizzo P, Robichaud K, Edwards B, Schumaker C, Kramer B, Johnson A. Oral antibiotic prophylaxis in patients with cancer: a double-blind randomized placebo-controlled trial. *J Pediatr*. 1983;102(1):125-133.

35. Horwitz R, Viscoli C, Berkman L, et al. Treatment adherence and risk of death after myocardial infarction. *Lancet*. 1990;336(8714):542-545.

36. Montori VM, Guyatt GH. The intention-to-treat principle. *CMAJ*. 2001;165(10):1339-1341.

37. Altman D, Gore S, Gardner M, Pocock S. Statistical guidelines for contributors to medical journals. In: Gardner M, Altman D, eds. *Statistics With Confidence Intervals and Statistical Guidelines*. London, England: British Medical Journal; 1989:83-100.

38. Guyatt G, Keller J, Singer J, Halcrow S, Newhouse M. Controlled trial of respiratory muscle training in chronic airflow limitation. *Thorax*. 1992;47(8):598-602.

39. Asymptomatic Carotid Atherosclerosis Study Group. Endarterectomy for asymptomatic carotid artery stenosis. *JAMA*. 1995;273(18):1421-1428.

40. Oxman A, Guyatt G. A consumer's guide to subgroup analysis. *Ann Intern Med*. 1992;116(1):78-84.

41. Guyatt G, Montori V, Devereaux P, Schunemann H, Bhandari M. Patients at the center: in our practice, and in our use of language. *ACP J Club*. 2004;140(1):A11-A12.

42. Echt D, Liebson P, Mitchell L, et al. Mortality and morbidity in patients receiving encainide, flecainide, or placebo: the Cardiac Arrhythmia Suppression Trial. *N Engl J Med*. 1991;324(12):781-788.

43. Cardiac Arrhythmia Suppression Trial II Investigators. Effect of antiarrhythmic agent moricizine on survival after myocardial infarction. *N Engl J Med*. 1992;327(4):227-233.

44. Ioannidis J, Lau J. Completeness of safety reporting in randomized trials: an evaluation of 7 medical areas. *JAMA*. 2001;285(4):437-443.

45. Carette S, Marcoux S, Treuchon R, et al. A controlled trial of corticosteroid injections into facet joints for chronic low back pain. *N Engl J Med.* 1991; 325(14):1002-1007.

46. Laupacis A, Sackett D, Roberts R. An assessment of clinically useful measures of the consequences of treatment. *N Engl J Med.* 1988; 318(26):1728-1733.

47. Malenka DJ, Baron JA, Johansen S, Wahrenberger JW, Ross JM. The framing effect of relative and absolute risk. *J Gen Intern Med.* 1993;8 (10):543-548.

DOES TREATMENT LOWER RISK? UNDERSTANDING THE RESULTS

Roman Jaeschke, Gordon Guyatt, Alexandra Barratt, Stephen Walter, and Deborah J. Cook

IN THIS CHAPTER:

When clinicians consider the results of clinical trials, they are interested in the association between a treatment and an *outcome*. This chapter will help you to understand and interpret study results related to outcomes that are either present or absent (*dichotomous*) for each patient, such as death, stroke, or myocardial infarction. A guide for teaching the *concepts* in this chapter is also available[1] (see http://www.cmaj.ca/cgi/data/171/4/353/DC1/1).

THE 2 × 2 TABLE

Table 7-1 depicts a 2 × 2 table that captures the information for a dichotomous outcome of a clinical trial.

TABLE 7-1

The 2 × 2 Table

	Outcome	
Exposure	**Yes**	**No**
Yes	a	b
No	c	d

Relative risk $= \dfrac{a/(a+b)}{c/(c+d)}$

Relative risk reduction $= \dfrac{c/(c+d) - a/(a+b)}{c/(c+d)}$

Risk difference[a] $= \dfrac{c}{c+d} - \dfrac{a}{a+b}$

Number needed to treat = 100/(risk difference expressed as %)

Odds ratio $= \dfrac{a/b}{c/d} = \dfrac{ad}{cb}$

[a]Also known as the absolute risk reduction.

TABLE 7-2

Results From a Randomized Trial of Endoscopic Sclerotherapy as Compared With Endoscopic Ligation for Bleeding Esophageal Varices[a]

Exposure	Outcome		Total
	Death	**Survival**	
Ligation	18	46	64
Sclerotherapy	29	36	65

Relative risk = (18/64) / (29/65) = 0.63

Relative risk reduction = 1 − 0.63 = 0.37

Risk difference = 0.446 − 0.281 = 0.165

Number needed to treat = 100/16.5 = 6

Odds ratio = (18/46) / (29/36) = 0.39 / 0.80 = 0.49

[a]Data from Stiegmann et al.[2]

For instance, in the course of a *randomized trial* comparing *mortality rates* in patients with bleeding esophageal varices that were controlled either by endoscopic ligation or by endoscopic sclerotherapy,[2] 18 of 64 participants assigned to ligation died, as did 29 of 65 patients assigned to sclerotherapy (Table 7-2).

THE RISK

The simplest measure of occurrence to understand is the *risk* (or *absolute risk*). We often refer to the risk of the adverse outcome in the *control group* as the *baseline risk* or the *control group risk*.

The risk of dying in the ligation group is 28% (18/64, or $[a/(a + b)]$), and the risk of dying in the sclerotherapy group is 45% (29/65, or $[c/(c + d)]$).

THE RISK DIFFERENCE (ABSOLUTE RISK REDUCTION)

One way of comparing 2 risks is by calculating the absolute difference between them. We refer to this difference as the *absolute risk reduction* (*ARR*) or the *risk difference* (*RD*). Algebraically, the formula for calculating the RD is $[c/(c + d)] - [a/(a + b)]$ (see Table 7-1). This measure of effect uses absolute rather than relative terms in looking at the proportion of patients who are spared the adverse outcome.

> In our example, the RD is $0.446 - 0.281$, or 0.165 (ie, an RD of 16.5%).

THE RELATIVE RISK

Another way to compare the risks in the 2 groups is to take their ratio; this is called the *relative risk* or *risk ratio* (*RR*). The RR tells us the proportion of the original risk (in this case, the risk of death with sclerotherapy) that is still present when patients receive the *experimental treatment* (in this case, ligation). From our 2×2 table, the formula for this calculation is $[a/(a + b)]/[c/(c + d)]$ (see Table 7-1).

> In our example, the RR of dying after receiving initial ligation vs sclerotherapy is 18/64 (the risk in the ligation group) divided by 29/65 (the risk in the sclerotherapy group), or 0.63. In everyday English, we would say the risk of death with ligation is about two-thirds that with sclerotherapy.

THE RELATIVE RISK REDUCTION

An alternative relative measure of treatment effectiveness is the *relative risk reduction* (*RRR*), an estimate of the proportion of baseline risk that is removed by the therapy. It may be calculated as $1 - RR$. One can also calculate the RRR by dividing the RD (amount of risk removed) by the absolute risk in the control group (see Table 7-1).

> In our bleeding varices example, where RR was 0.63, the RRR is thus $1 - 0.63$ (or 16.5% divided by 44.6%, the risk in the sclerotherapy group)—either way, it comes to 0.37. In other words, ligation decreases the risk of death by about a third compared with sclerotherapy.

THE ODDS RATIO

Instead of looking at the risk of an event, we could estimate the odds of having vs not having an event. When considering the effects of therapy, you usually will not go far wrong if you interpret the *odds ratio* (*OR*) as equivalent to the RR. The exception is when event rates are very high—for instance, more than 40% of control patients experience myocardial infarction or death.

RELATIVE RISK VS RISK DIFFERENCE: WHY THE FUSS?

Failing to distinguish between the OR and the RR when interpreting randomized trial results will seldom mislead you; you must, however, distinguish between the RR and the RD. The reason is that the RR is generally far larger than the RD, and presentations of results in the form of RR (or RRR) can convey a misleading message. Reducing a patient's risk by 50% sounds impressive. That may, however, represent a reduction in risk from 2% to 1%. The corresponding 1% RD sounds considerably less impressive.

As depicted in Figure 7-1, consider a treatment that is administered to 3 different subpopulations of patients and which, in each case, decreases the risk by $1/3$ (RRR, 0.33; RR, 0.67). When administered to a subpopulation with a 30% risk of dying, treatment reduces

FIGURE 7-1

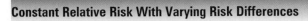

Constant Relative Risk With Varying Risk Differences

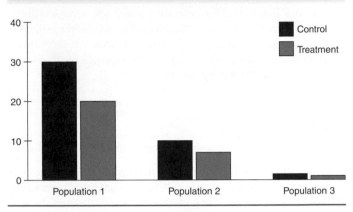

the risk to 20%. When administered to a population with a 10% risk of dying, treatment reduces the risk to 6.7%. In the third population, treatment reduces the risk of dying from 1% to 0.67%.

Although treatment reduces the risk of dying by a third in each population, this piece of information is not adequate to fully capture the impact of treatment. What if the treatment under consideration is a toxic cancer chemotherapy in which 10% of those treated experience severe adverse effects? Under these circumstances, we would probably not recommend the treatment to most patients in the lowest risk group in Figure 7-1, whose RD is only 0.3%. We would certainly explain the benefits and risks of treatment to the intermediate population, those with an absolute reduction in risk of death of about 3%. In the highest risk population with an absolute benefit of 10%, we could confidently recommend the treatment to most patients.

We suggest that you consider the RRR in the light of your patient's baseline risk. For instance, you might expect an RRR of approximately 30% in vascular events in patients with possible cardiovascular disease with administration of statins. You would view this RRR differently in a 40-year-old female normotensive nondiabetic nonsmoker with a mildly elevated LDL (low-density lipoprotein) (5-year risk of a cardiovascular event of approximately 2%, ARR of about 0.7%) and a 70-year-old hypertensive diabetic smoker (5-year risk of 30%, ARR of 10%). All this assumes a constant RRR across risk groups; fortunately, a more or less constant RRR is usually the case, and we suggest you make that assumption unless there is evidence that suggests it is incorrect.[3-5]

THE NUMBER NEEDED TO TREAT

One can also express the impact of treatment by the number of patients one would need to treat to prevent an adverse event, the *number needed to treat* (*NNT*).[6] Table 7-2 shows that the risk of dying in the ligation group is 28.1%; and in the sclerotherapy group, it is 44.6%, an RD of 16.5%. If treating 100 patients results in avoiding 16.5 events, how many patients do we need to treat to avoid 1 event? The answer, 100 divided by 16.5, or approximately 6, is the NNT.

Given knowledge of the baseline risk and RRR, a *nomogram* presents another way of arriving at the NNT (Figure 7-2).[7] NNT calculation always implies a given time of *follow-up* (ie, do we need to treat 50 patients for 1 year or 5 years to prevent an event?). When trials with long follow-ups are analyzed by survival methods (see following), there are a variety of ways of calculating the NNT. The impact of these different methods will, however, almost never be important.[8]

Assuming a constant RRR, the NNT is inversely related to the proportion of patients in the control group who have an adverse event. If the risk of an adverse event doubles (for example, if we deal with patients at a higher risk of death than those included in the clinical trial), we need to treat only half as many patients to prevent an adverse event; if the risk decreases by a factor of 4 (patients are younger, have less *comorbidity* than those in the study), we will have to treat 4 times as many people.

FIGURE 7-2

Nomogram for Calculating the Number Needed to Treat

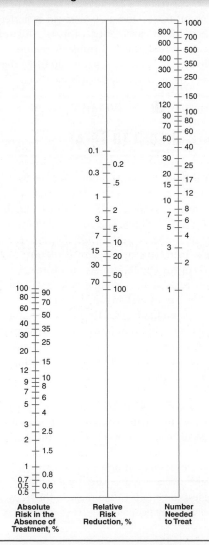

Absolute Risk in the Absence of Treatment, %	Relative Risk Reduction, %	Number Needed to Treat

Reproduced from Chatellier,[7] with permission from the BMJ Publishing Group.

The NNT is also inversely related to the RRR. With the same baseline risk, a more effective treatment with twice the RRR will reduce the NNT by half. If the RRR with 1 treatment is only a quarter of that achieved by an alternative strategy, the NNT will be 4 times greater.

Table 7-3 presents hypothetical data that illustrate these relationships.

THE NUMBER NEEDED TO HARM

Clinicians can calculate the *number needed to harm* (*NNH*) in a similar way. If you expect 5 of 100 patients to become fatigued when taking a β-blocker for a year, you will have to treat 20 patients to cause 1 to become tired; and the NNH is 20.

TABLE 7-3

Relationship Among the Baseline Risk, the Relative Risk Reduction, and the Number Needed to Treat[a]

Control Group Risk	Experi-mental Group Risk	Relative Risk, %	Relative Risk Reduc-tion, %	Risk Difference	Number Needed to Treat
0.02	0.01	50	50	0.01	100
0.4	0.2	50	50	0.2	5
0.04	0.02	50	50	0.02	50
0.04	0.03	75	25	0.01	100
0.4	0.3	75	25	0.1	10
0.01	0.005	50	50	0.005	200

[a]Relative risk = experimental group risk/control group risk; relative risk reduction = 1 – relative risk; risk difference = control group risk – experimental group risk; number needed to treat = 1/risk difference (in decimal).

CONFIDENCE INTERVALS

We have presented all of the measures of association of the treatment with ligation vs sclerotherapy as if they represented the true effect. The results of any experiment, however, represent only an estimate of the truth. The true effect of treatment may be somewhat greater—or less—than what we observed. The *confidence interval* tells us, within the bounds of plausibility, how much greater or smaller the true effect is likely to be (see Chapter 8, Confidence Intervals).

SURVIVAL DATA

Analysis of a 2×2 table implies an examination of the data at a specific point in time. This analysis is satisfactory if we are looking for events that occur within relatively short periods and if all patients have the same duration of follow-up. In longer-term studies, however, we are interested not only in the total number of events but also in their timing. For instance, we may focus on whether therapy for patients with a uniformly fatal condition (unresectable lung cancer, for example) delays death.

When the timing of events is important, investigators could present the results in the form of several 2×2 tables constructed at different points of time after the study began. For example, Table 7-2 represents the situation after the study was finished. Similar tables could be constructed describing the fate of all patients available for analysis after their enrollment in the trial for 1 week, 1 month, 3 months, or whatever time we choose to examine. The analysis of accumulated data that takes into account the timing of events is called *survival analysis*. Do not infer from the name, however, that the analysis is restricted to deaths; in fact, any dichotomous outcome occurring over time will qualify.

The *survival curve* of a group of patients describes their status at different times after a defined starting point.[9] In Figure 7-3, we show

FIGURE 7-3

Survival Curves for Ligation and Sclerotherapy

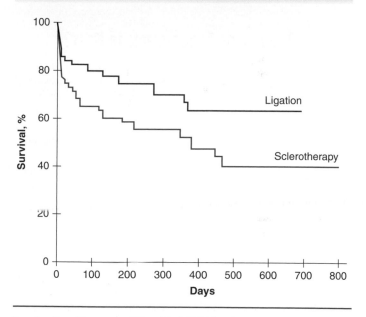

the survival curve from the bleeding varices trial. Because the investigators followed some patients for a longer time, the survival curve extends beyond the mean follow-up of about 10 months. At some point, prediction becomes very imprecise because there are few patients remaining to estimate the *probability* of survival. Confidence intervals around the survival curves capture the precision of the estimate.

Even if the true RR, or RRR, is constant throughout the duration of follow-up, the play of chance will ensure that the *point estimates* differ. Ideally then, we would estimate the overall RR by applying an average, weighted for the number of patients available, for the entire survival experience. Statistical methods allow just such an estimate. The weighted RR over the entire study is known as the *hazard ratio*.

WHICH MEASURE OF ASSOCIATION IS BEST?

As evidence-based practitioners, we must decide which measure of association deserves our focus. Does it matter? The answer is yes. The same results, when presented in different ways, may lead to different treatment decisions.[10-14] For example, Forrow et al[10] demonstrated that clinicians were less inclined to treat patients after presentation of trial results as the absolute change in the outcome compared with the relative change in the outcome. In a similar study, Naylor et al[11] found that clinicians rated the effectiveness of an intervention lower when events were presented in absolute terms rather than using RRR. Moreover, clinicians offered lower effectiveness ratings when they viewed results expressed in terms of NNT than when they saw the same data as RRRs or ARRs. The pharmaceutic industry's awareness of this phenomenon may be responsible for their propensity to present physicians with treatment-associated RRRs.

Patients are as susceptible as clinicians to how results are communicated.[7,15-17] In one study, when researchers presented patients with a hypothetical scenario of life-threatening illness, the patients were more likely to choose a treatment described in terms of RRR than in terms of the corresponding ARR.[15]

Considering how our interpretations differ with data presentations, we are best advised to consider all the data (either as a 2 × 2 table or as a survival analysis) and then reflect on both the relative and the absolute figures. As you examine the results, you will find that if you can estimate your patient's baseline risk, knowing how well the treatment works—expressed as an RR or RRR—allows you to estimate the patient's risk with treatment. Considering the RD— the difference between the risk with and without treatment—and its reciprocal, the NNT, in an individual patient, will be most useful in guiding the treatment decision.

References

1. Barratt A, Wyer PC, Hatala R, et al. Tips for learners of evidence-based medicine, 1: relative risk reduction, absolute risk reduction and number needed to treat. *CMAJ.* 2004;171(4:online-1 to online-8):353-358.

2. Stiegmann GV, Goff JS, Michaletz-Onody PA, et al. Endoscopic sclerotherapy as compared with endoscopic ligation for bleeding esophageal varices. *N Engl J Med.* 1992;326(23):1527-1532.

3. Deeks JJ. Issues in the selection of a summary statistic for meta-analysis of clinical trials with binary outcomes. *Stat Med.* 2002;21(11):1575-1600.

4. Schmid CH, Lau J, McIntosh MW, Cappelleri JC. An empirical study of the effect of the control rate as a predictor of treatment efficacy in meta-analysis of clinical trials. *Stat Med.* 1998;17(17):1923-1942.

5. Furukawa TA, Guyatt GH, Griffith LE. Can we individualize the "number needed to treat"? an empirical study of summary effect measures in meta-analyses. *Int J Epidemiol.* 2002;31(1):72-76.

6. Laupacis A, Sackett DL, Roberts RS. An assessment of clinically useful measures of the consequences of treatment. *N Engl J Med.* 1988;318(26):1728-1733.

7. Chatellier G, Zapletal E, Lemaitre D, Menard J, Degoulet P. The number needed to treat: a clinically useful nomogram in its proper context. *BMJ.* 1996;312(7028):426-429.

8. Barratt AW, Guyatt G, Simpsons J. NNT for studies with long-term follow-up. *CMAJ.* 2005;172(5):613-615.

9. Coldman AJ, Elwood JM. Examining survival data. *CMAJ.* 1979;121(8):1065-1068, 1071.

10. Forrow L, Taylor WC, Arnold RM. Absolutely relative: how research results are summarized can affect treatment decisions. *Am J Med.* 1992;92(2):121-124.

11. Naylor CD, Chen E, Strauss B. Measured enthusiasm: does the method of reporting trial results alter perceptions of therapeutic effectiveness? *Ann Intern Med.* 1992;117(11):916-921.

12. Hux JE, Levinton CM, Naylor CD. Prescribing propensity: influence of life-expectancy gains and drug costs. *J Gen Intern Med.* 1994;9(4):195-201.

13. Redelmeier DA, Tversky A. Discrepancy between medical decisions for individual patients and for groups. *N Engl J Med.* 1990;322(16):1162-1164.

14. Bobbio M, Demichelis B, Giustetto G. Completeness of reporting trial results: effect on physicians' willingness to prescribe. *Lancet.* 1994;343(8907):1209-1211.

15. Malenka DJ, Baron JA, Johansen S, Wahrenberger JW, Ross JM. The framing effect of relative and absolute risk. *J Gen Intern Med.* 1993;8(10):543-548.

16. McNeil BJ, Pauker SG, Sox HC Jr, Tversky A. On the elicitation of preferences for alternative therapies. *N Engl J Med.* 1982;306(21):1259-1262.

17. Hux JE, Naylor CD. Communicating the benefits of chronic preventive therapy: does the format of efficacy data determine patients' acceptance of treatment? *Med Decis Making.* 1995;15(2):152-157.

CONFIDENCE INTERVALS

Gordon Guyatt, Stephen Walter, Deborah J. Cook,
Peter Wyer, and Roman Jaeschke

IN THIS CHAPTER:

Hypothesis testing involves estimating the probability that observed results would have occurred by chance if a *null hypothesis*, which most commonly states that there is no difference between a treatment condition and a control condition, were true. Health researchers and medical educators have increasingly recognized the limitations of hypothesis testing; consequently, an alternative approach, estimation, is becoming more popular. Several authors[1-5]—including ourselves, in an article on which this chapter is based[6]—have outlined the *concepts* that we will introduce here; and you can use their discussions to supplement our presentation.

HOW SHOULD WE TREAT PATIENTS WITH HEART FAILURE? A PROBLEM IN INTERPRETING STUDY RESULTS

In a *blinded randomized controlled trial* of 804 men with heart failure, investigators compared treatment with enalapril to that with a combination of hydralazine and nitrates.[7] In the *follow-up* period, which ranged from 6 months to 5.7 years, 132 of 403 patients (33%) assigned to receive enalapril died, as did 153 of 401 patients (38%) assigned to receive hydralazine and nitrates. The *P* value associated with the difference in mortality is .11.

Looking at this study as an exercise in hypothesis testing and adopting the usual 5% risk of obtaining a false-positive result, we would conclude that chance remains a plausible explanation of the apparent differences between groups. We would classify this as a *negative study*; ie, we would conclude that no important difference existed between the treatment and *control groups*.

The investigators also conducted an analysis that compared not only the proportion of patients surviving at the end of the study but also the time pattern of the deaths occurring in both groups. This *survival analysis*, which generally is more sensitive than the test of the difference in proportions (see Chapter 7, Does Treatment Lower Risk? Understanding the Results), showed a nonsignificant *P* value of .08, a result that leads to the same conclusion as the simpler analysis that focused on relative proportions at the end of the study. The authors also tell us that the *P* value associated with differences in mortality at 2 years (a point predetermined to be a major *endpoint* of the trial) was significant at .016.

At this point, one might excuse clinicians who feel a little confused. Ask yourself, is this a *positive trial* dictating use of an angiotensin-converting enzyme (ACE) inhibitor instead of the combination of hydralazine and nitrates, or is it a negative study, showing no difference between the 2 regimens and leaving the choice of drugs open?

SOLVING THE PROBLEM: WHAT ARE CONFIDENCE INTERVALS?

How can clinicians deal with the limitations of hypothesis testing and resolve the confusion? The solution involves posing 2 questions: (1) What is the single value most likely to represent the true difference between experimental and control? and (2) Given the observed difference between experimental and control, what is the plausible range of differences between them within which the true difference might actually lie? *Confidence intervals* provide an answer to this second question. Before applying confidence intervals to resolve the issue of enalapril vs hydralazine and nitrates in patients with heart failure, we will illustrate the use of confidence intervals with a thought experiment.

Imagine a series of 5 trials (of equal duration but different sample sizes) wherein investigators have experimented with treating patients with a particular condition (elevated low-density-lipoprotein cholesterol) to determine whether a drug (a novel cholesterol-lowering agent) would work better than a *placebo* to *prevent* strokes (Table 8-1). The smallest trial enrolled only 8 patients, and the largest enrolled 2000 patients.

TABLE 8-1

Relative Risk Reduction Observed in 5 Successively Larger Hypothetical Trials

Control Group Risk	Experimental Group Risk	Relative Risk, %	Relative Risk Reduction, %[a]
2/4	1/4	50	50
10/20	5/20	50	50
20/40	10/40	50	50
50/100	25/100	50	50
500/1000	250/1000	50	50

[a]Expressing event rates as a fraction, if the control group risk were 3/4 and the experimental group risk were 1/4 or 2/4, the relative risk reduction would be [(3/4) – (1/4)]/(3/4) = 2/3 or [(3/4) – (2/4)]/(3/4) = 1/3, respectively. Expressing event rates as percentage, if the control group risk were 75% and the experimental group risk were 25% or 50%, the relative risk reduction would be (75% – 25%)/75% = 67% or (75% – 50%)/75% = 33%, respectively.

Reprinted from Montori et al,[6] by permission of the publisher. Copyright © 2005, Canadian Medical Association.

> Now imagine that all the trials showed a *relative risk reduction (RRR)* for the treatment group of 50% (meaning that patients in the drug treatment group were 50% as likely as those in the placebo group to have a stroke). In each trial, how confident can we be that the true value of the RRR is *patient-important*?[8] If you were looking at the studies individually, which ones would lead your patients to use the treatment?

Most clinicians know intuitively that we can be more confident in the results of a larger vs a smaller trial. Why is this? In the absence of *bias* or *systematic error*, one can interpret the trial as providing an estimate of the true magnitude of effect that would occur if all possible eligible patients had participated. When only a few patients participate, chance may lead to a best estimate of the *treatment effect*—the *point estimate*— that is far removed from the true value. Confidence intervals are a numeric measure of the range within which such variation is likely to occur. The 95% confidence intervals that we often see in biomedical publications represent the range in which we can be 95% certain of finding the underlying true treatment effect.

To gain a better appreciation of confidence intervals, go back to Table 8-1 (do not look at Table 8-2 yet!) and take a guess at what you think the confidence intervals might be for the 5 trials presented. In a moment, you will see how your estimates compare with the actual calculated 95% confidence intervals, but for now, try figuring out an interval that you think would be intuitive.

Now consider the first trial, in which 2 of 4 patients receiving the control intervention and 1 of 4 patients receiving the experimental treatment intervention have a stroke. The risk in the experimental group was thus half of that in the control group, giving a *relative risk (RR)* of 50% and an RRR of 50%.

Would you be ready to recommend this treatment to a patient in view of the substantial RRR? Before you answer this, consider whether it is plausible that, with so few patients in the study, we could have just been lucky in our sample and the true treatment effect could really be a 50% increase in RR. In other words, is it plausible that the true *event rate* in the group that received treatment was 3 of 4 instead of 1 of 4? If you accept that this large, harmful effect may represent the underlying truth, would an RRR of 90% (ie, a large benefit of treatment) also be consistent with the experimental data in these few patients? To the extent that these suggestions are plausible, we can intuitively create a range of plausible truth of −50% to 90% surrounding the RRR of 50% that we actually observed in the study.

Now do this for each of the other 4 trials. In the trial with 20 patients in the experimental group and 20 in the control group, 10 of 20 patients in the control group had a stroke, as did 5 of 20 patients in the experimental group. The RR and RRR are again 50%. Do you still consider plausible that the true event rate in the experimental group is really 15 of 20 rather than 5 of 20? If not, what about 12 of 20? The latter would yield an increase in the RR of 20%. A true RRR of 90% may still remain plausible, given the observed results and numbers of patients involved. In short, given

TABLE 8-2

Confidence Intervals Around the Relative Risk Reduction for the Hypothetical Results of 5 Successively Larger Trials

Control Group Risk	Experimental Group Risk	Relative Risk, %	Relative Risk Reduction, %	Intuitive Confidence Interval, %	Calculated 95% Confidence Interval Around the RRR, %
2/4	1/4	50	50	−50 to 90	−174 to 92
10/20	5/20	50	50	−20 to 90	−14 to 79.5
20/40	10/40	50	50	0 to 90	9.5 to 73.4
50/100	25/100	50	50	20 to 80	26.8 to 66.4
500/1000	250/1000	50	50	40 to 60	43.5 to 55.9

Reprinted from Montori et al,[6] by permission of the publisher. Copyright © 2005, Canadian Medical Association.

this larger number of patients and lower chance of a bad sample, your range of plausible truth around the observed RRR of 50% might be narrower, perhaps from –20% (an RR increase of 20%) to a 90% RRR.

For the larger and larger trials, you could provide similar intuitively derived confidence intervals. We have done this in Table 8-2, and also provided the 95% confidence intervals (calculated using a statistical program). You can see that, in some instances, we intuitively overestimated or underestimated the calculated intervals.

Confidence intervals inform clinicians about the range within which, given the trial data, the true treatment effect might plausibly lie. More precision (narrower confidence intervals) results from larger sample sizes and consequently larger number of events. Statisticians (and clinician-friendly statistical software) can calculate 95% confidence intervals around any estimate of treatment effect.

USING CONFIDENCE INTERVALS TO INTERPRET THE RESULTS OF CLINICAL TRIALS

How do confidence intervals help us understand the results of the trial of vasodilators in patients with heart failure? Throughout the entire study, the mortality in the ACE inhibitor arm was 33% and in the hydralazine plus nitrate group it was 38%, an *absolute difference* of 5% and an RR of 0.86. The 5% absolute difference and the 14% RRR represent our best single estimate of the mortality benefit from using an ACE inhibitor. The 95% confidence interval around the RRR works out to –3.5% to 29% (that is, 3.5% RRR with hydralazine and nitrates, to a 29% RRR with the ACE inhibitor).

How can we now interpret the study results? We can conclude that patients offered ACE inhibitors will most likely (but not certainly) die later than patients offered hydralazine and nitrates—but the magnitude of the difference may be either trivial or quite large, and there remains the possibility of a marginally lower mortality with the hydralazine-nitrate regimen.

Using the confidence interval avoids the yes/no dichotomy of hypothesis testing. It also obviates the need to argue whether the study should be considered positive or negative. One can conclude that, all else being equal, an ACE inhibitor is the appropriate choice for patients with heart failure, but the strength of this inference is weak. Toxicity, expense, and *evidence* from other studies would all bear on the final treatment decision (see Chapter 15, How to Use a Patient Management Recommendation). Because a number of large randomized trials have now shown a mortality benefit from ACE inhibitors in patients with heart failure,[9] one can confidently recommend this class of agents as the treatment of choice. Another study has suggested that for black patients, the hydralazine-nitrate combination offers additional mortality reduction beyond ACE inhibitors.[10]

INTERPRETING APPARENTLY "NEGATIVE" TRIALS

Another example of the use of confidence intervals in interpreting study results comes from a randomized trial of low vs high positive end expiratory pressure (PEEP) in patients with adult respiratory distress syndrome.[11] Of 273 patients in the low-PEEP group, 24.9% died; of 276 in the high-PEEP group, 27.5% died. The point estimate from these results is a 2.6% *absolute risk increase* in deaths in the high-PEEP group.

This trial of more than 500 patients might appear to exclude any possible benefit from high PEEP. The 95% confidence interval on the absolute difference of 2.6% in favor of low PEEP, however, is from 10.0% in favor of low PEEP to 4.7% in favor of high PEEP. Were it true that 4.7% of the patients who would have died if given low PEEP would survive if treated with high PEEP, all patients would want to receive the high-PEEP strategy. This would mean one would need to treat only 21 patients to prevent a premature death. One can thus conclude that the trial has not excluded a patient-important benefit and, in that sense, was not large enough.

This example emphasizes that many patients must participate if trials are to generate precise estimates of treatment effects. In addition, it illustrates why we recommend that, whenever possible, clinicians turn to systematic reviews that pool data from the most valid studies.

When you see an apparently *negative trial* (one with a *P* value greater than .05 that, using conventional criteria, fails to exclude the null hypothesis that treatment and control interventions do not differ), you can focus on the upper end of the confidence interval (that is, the end that suggests the largest benefit from treatment). If the upper boundary of the confidence interval excludes any important benefit of treatment, you can conclude that the trial is definitively negative. If, on the other hand, the confidence interval includes an important benefit, the possibility should not be ruled out that the treatment still might be worthwhile.

This logic of the negative trial is crucial in the interpretation of studies designed to help determine whether we should substitute a treatment that is less expensive, easier to administer, or less toxic for an existing treatment. In such *noninferiority studies*, we will be ready to make the substitution only if we are sure that the standard treatment does not have important additional benefits beyond the less expensive or more convenient substitute.[12-15] We will be confident that we have excluded the possibility of important additional benefits of the standard treatment if the boundary of the confidence interval representing the largest plausible treatment effect is below our threshold.

INTERPRETING APPARENTLY "POSITIVE" TRIALS

How can confidence intervals be informative in a positive trial (one that, yielding a P value less than .05, makes chance an unlikely explanation for observed differences between treatments)? In a blinded trial in patients with vascular disease, 19 185 patients were randomized to clopidogrel or aspirin. Patients receiving clopidogrel experienced a 5.32% annual risk of ischemic stroke, myocardial infarction, or vascular death vs 5.83% with aspirin, an RRR of 8.7% in favor of clopidogrel (95% confidence interval, 0.3%-16.5%; $P = .043$). In absolute terms, the difference between treatments is 0.5%, with a 95% confidence interval of 0.02%—that is, 2 in 10 000—to 0.9%, or just less than 1 in 100. For the average patient, one could argue whether the point estimate of 0.5% absolute difference—a *number needed to treat* (*NNT*) of 200—represents an important difference. Few patients are likely to find the lower boundary of the confidence interval, representing an NNT of 5000, an important difference. This trial does not establish clopidogrel's superiority over aspirin. The sample size—almost 20 000 patients—was insufficient to provide a definitive answer.

WAS THE TRIAL LARGE ENOUGH?

As implied in our discussion to this point, confidence intervals provide a way of answering the question: was the trial large enough? We illustrate the approach in Figure 8-1. In this figure, we present the results of 4 randomized trials. Although most forest plots (visual plots of trial results) focus on RR or odds ratios, Figure 8-1 presents the results in absolute terms. Thus, the solid vertical line in the center of the figure represents a *risk difference* (*RD*) (or *absolute risk reduction*) of zero, when the experimental and control groups have the same mortality. Values to the left of the vertical line represent

FIGURE 8-1

When Is Trial Sample Size Sufficiently Large? Four Hypothetical Trial Results

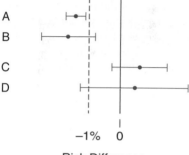

$$-1\% \quad 0$$

Risk Difference

For the medical condition under investigation, a risk difference of –1% (broken line) is the smallest benefit that patients would consider important enough to warrant undergoing treatment.

Reprinted from Montori et al,[6] by permission of the publisher. Copyright © 2005, Canadian Medical Association.

results in which the treated group had a lower mortality than the control group. Values to the right of the vertical line represent results in which the treated group fared worse and had a higher mortality rate than the control group.

Assume that the treatment carries sufficient toxicity or risk such that, in each case, patients would choose treatment only if the RD were 1% or greater. That is, if the reduction in death rates were greater than 1%, patients would consider it worth enduring the toxicity and risk of treatment, but if the reduction in event rates were less than 1%, they would not. The broken line in Figure 8-1 represents the threshold reduction in death rates of 1%.

Now consider trial A: would you recommend this therapy to your patients if the point estimate represented the truth? What if the upper boundary of the confidence interval represented the truth? What about the lower boundary?

For all 3, the answer is yes, given that 1% is the smallest patient-important difference, and all suggest a benefit of greater than 1%. Thus, the trial is definitive and provides a strong inference about the treatment decision.

In the case of trial B, would your patients choose to take the treatment if either the point estimate or the upper boundary of the confidence interval represented the true effect? The answer is yes, the patients would, for the reduction in death rate would be greater than the 1% threshold. What about the lower boundary? The answer here is no, for the effect is less than the smallest difference that patients would consider large enough to take the treatment. Although trial B shows a positive result (ie, the confidence interval excludes an effect of zero), the sample size was inadequate and yielded a result that remains compatible with risk reductions below the minimal patient-important difference.

For negative studies, those that fail to exclude a true treatment effect of zero, you should focus on the other end of the confidence interval, that which represents the largest plausible treatment effect consistent with the trial data. You should consider whether that upper boundary of the confidence interval falls below the smallest difference that patients might consider important. If so, the sample size is adequate and the trial is negative and definitive (Figure 8-1, trial C). If the boundary representing the largest plausible effect exceeds the smallest patient-important difference, then the trial is not definitive and more trials with larger sample sizes are needed (Figure 8-1, trial D).[6]

We can state our message as follows: In a positive trial establishing that the effect of treatment is greater than zero, look to the lower boundary of the confidence interval to determine whether sample size has been adequate. If this lower boundary—the smallest plausible treatment effect compatible with the data—is greater than the smallest difference that you consider important, the sample size is adequate and the trial is definitive. If the lower boundary is less than this smallest important difference, the trial is nondefinitive and further trials are required.

In a negative trial, look to the upper boundary of the confidence interval to determine whether sample size has been adequate. If this upper boundary, the largest treatment effect plausibly compatible with the data, is less than the smallest difference that you consider important, the sample size is adequate and the trial is definitively negative. If the upper boundary exceeds the smallest important difference, there may still be an important positive treatment effect, the trial is nondefinitive, and further trials are required.

Acknowledgment

Portions of this material were previously published from Montori et al.[6]

References

1. Simon R. Confidence intervals for reporting results of clinical trials. *Ann Intern Med.* 1986;105(3):429-435.

2. Gardner M. *Statistics With Confidence: Confidence Intervals and Statistical Guidelines*. London, England: BMJ Publishing Group; 1989.

3. Bulpitt CJ. Confidence intervals. *Lancet.* 1987;1(8531):494-497.

4. Pocock SJ, Hughes MD. Estimation issues in clinical trials and overviews. *Stat Med.* 1990;9(6):657-671.

5. Braitman LE. Confidence intervals assess both clinical significance and statistical significance. *Ann Intern Med.* 1991;114(6):515-517.

6. Montori VM, Kleinbart J, Newman TB, et al. Tips for learners of evidence-based medicine, 2: measures of precision (confidence intervals). *CMAJ.* 2004;171(6):611-615.

7. Cohn JN, Johnson G, Ziesche S, et al. A comparison of enalapril with hydralazine-isosorbide dinitrate in the treatment of chronic congestive heart failure. *N Engl J Med.* 1991;325(5):303-310.

8. Guyatt G, Montori V, Devereaux PJ, Schunemann H, Bhandari M. Patients at the center: in our practice, and in our use of language. *ACP J Club.* 2004;140(1):A11-A12.

9. Garg R, Yusuf S. Overview of randomized trials of angiotensin-converting enzyme inhibitors on mortality and morbidity in patients with heart failure: Collaborative Group on ACE Inhibitor Trials. *JAMA.* 1995;273(18):1450-1456.

10. Taylor AL, Ziesche S, Yancy C, et al. Combination of isosorbide dinitrate and hydralazine in blacks with heart failure. *N Engl J Med.* 2004;351 (20):2049-2057.

11. Brower RG, Lanken PN, MacIntyre N, et al. Higher versus lower positive end-expiratory pressures in patients with the acute respiratory distress syndrome. *N Engl J Med.* 2004;351(4):327-336.

12. D'Agostino RB Sr, Massaro JM, Sullivan LM. Non-inferiority trials: design concepts and issues—the encounters of academic consultants in statistics. *Stat Med.* 2003;22(2):169-186.

13. Gotzsche PC. Lessons from and cautions about noninferiority and equivalence randomized trials. *JAMA.* 2006;295(10):1172-1174.

14. Piaggio G, Elbourne DR, Altman DG, Pocock SJ, Evans SJ. Reporting of noninferiority and equivalence randomized trials: an extension of the CONSORT statement. *JAMA.* 2006;295(10):1152-1160.

15. Le Henanff A, Giraudeau B, Baron G, Ravaud P. Quality of reporting of noninferiority and equivalence randomized trials. *JAMA.* 2006;295(10):1147-1151.

HARM (OBSERVATIONAL STUDIES)

Mitchell Levine, John Ioannidis, Ted Haines, and Gordon Guyatt

IN THIS CHAPTER:

Was Follow-up Sufficiently Long?

Is the Exposure Similar to What Might Occur in My Patient?

What Is the Magnitude of the Risk?

Are There Any Benefits That Offset the Risks Associated With Exposure?

Clinical Resolution

CLINICAL SCENARIO

Does Soy Milk (or Soy Formula) Increase the Risk of Developing Peanut Allergy in Children?

You are a general practitioner with a 29-year-old patient who is 8 months pregnant with her second child. Her first child, who is now 3 years old, had demonstrated an intolerance to cow's milk as an infant. He was switched to soy formula, and then soy milk, which he subsequently tolerated very well. At age 2 years, cow's milk was reintroduced without any problems, and he has been receiving cow's milk since. She was planning to start feeding her next child soy formula at birth but heard from a neighbor that it can increase the risk of peanut allergy in her child, a potentially serious and lifelong disease. She asks for your advice on the topic. Because you are not particularly familiar with this issue, you inform your patient that you will examine the evidence and discuss your findings with her when she returns for her next prenatal visit in 1 week.

FINDING THE EVIDENCE

You formulate the relevant question: In infants, what is the association between *exposure* to soy milk and the subsequent development of peanut allergy? Searching Ovid (MEDLINE) with the terms "peanut" AND "soy" AND "allergy" AND "risk," you identify 12 articles. One article appears to be particularly relevant to your target: factors associated with the development of peanut allergy in childhood.[1] You print a copy of the abstract and then arrange to obtain a copy of the full-text article from your local hospital library.

The article describes a case-control study that used a geographically defined cohort of 13 971 preschool children. The investigators identified children with a convincing history of peanut allergy who reacted to a blinded peanut challenge. They collected detailed information from the children's parents and from 2 groups of control parents (a random sample from the geographically defined cohort and from a subgroup of children from the cohort who had eczema in the first 6 months of life and whose mothers had a history of eczema).

Table 9-1 presents our usual 3-step approach to using an article about harm from the medical literature to guide your practice. You will find these criteria useful for a variety of issues involving concerns of etiology or risk factors in which a potentially harmful exposure cannot be randomly assigned. These *observational studies* involve using either cohort or case-control designs.

ARE THE RESULTS VALID?

Clinicians often encounter patients who face potentially harmful exposures either to medical interventions or environmental agents. These circumstances give rise to important questions. Are pregnant women at increased risk of miscarriage if they work in front of video display terminals? Do vasectomies increase the risk of prostate cancer? Do changes in health care policies lead to harmful outcomes? When examining these questions, health care providers and administrators must evaluate the validity of the data, the strength of the association between the assumed cause and the adverse outcome, and the relevance to patients in their domain.

In answering any clinical question, our first goal should be to identify any existing *systematic review* of the topic that can provide a

TABLE 9-1

Users' Guides for an Article About Harm

Are the results valid?

In a cohort study, aside from the exposure of interest, did the exposed and control groups start and finish with the same risk for the outcome?

- Were patients similar for prognostic factors that are known to be associated with the outcome (or did statistical adjustment level the playing field)?
- Were the circumstances and methods for detecting the outcome similar?
- Was the follow-up sufficiently complete?

In a case-control study, did the cases and control group have the same risk (chance) for being exposed in the past?

- Were cases and controls similar with respect to the indication or circumstances that would lead to exposure?
- Were the circumstances and methods for determining exposure similar for cases and controls?

What are the results?

- How strong is the association between exposure and outcome?
- How precise was the estimate of the risk?

How can I apply the result to patient care?

- Were the study patients similar to the patient in my practice?
- Was follow-up sufficiently long?
- Is the exposure similar to what might occur in my patient?
- What is the magnitude of the risk?
- Are there any benefits that are known to be associated with exposure?

summary of the highest-quality available evidence (see Chapter 14, Summarizing the Evidence). Interpreting such a *review* requires an understanding of the rules of evidence for individual or *primary studies, randomized controlled trials (RCTs)*, and observational studies. The tests for judging the validity of observational study results will help you decide whether exposed and control groups (or cases and controls) began and finished the study with sufficient similarities that we obtain a minimally biased assessment of the influence of exposure on outcome (see Chapter 5, Why Study Results Mislead: Bias and Random Error).

RCTs provide less biased estimates of potentially harmful effects than other study designs because randomization is the best way to ensure that groups are balanced with respect to both known and unknown determinants of the outcome (see Chapter 6, Therapy). Although investigators conduct RCTs to determine whether therapeutic agents are beneficial, they should also look for harmful effects and may sometimes make surprising discoveries about the negative effects of the intervention on their primary outcomes.[2]

There are 3 reasons why RCTs may not be helpful for determining whether a putative harmful agent truly has deleterious effects. First, we would consider it unethical to randomize patients to exposures that we anticipate might result in harmful effects without benefit. Second, we are often concerned about rare and serious adverse effects that may become evident only after tens of thousands of patients have consumed a medication for a period of years. Even a very large RCT[3] failed to detect an association between clopidogrel and thrombotic thrombocytopenic purpura, which appeared in a subsequent observational study.[4] RCTs specifically addressing adverse effects may be feasible for adverse event rates as low as 1%.[5,6] But the RCTs that we need to explore harmful events occurring in less than 1 in 100 exposed patients are logistically difficult and often prohibitively expensive because of huge sample size and lengthy follow-up. Meta-analyses may be very helpful when the event rates are very low.[7] Across almost 2000 systematic reviews, however, only 25 reviews had large-scale data on 4000 or more randomized subjects regarding well-defined harms that might be associated with the assessed interventions.[8] Third, RCTs often fail to adequately information on harm.[9]

Given that clinicians will not find RCTs to answer most questions about harm, they must understand the alternative strategies used to minimize *bias*. This requires a familiarity with observational study designs, which we will now describe (Table 9-2). There are 2 main types of observational studies, cohort and case-control. In a cohort study, the

TABLE 9-2

Directions of Inquiry and Key Methodologic Strengths and Weaknesses for Different Study Designs

Design	Starting Point	Assessment	Strengths	Weaknesses
Randomized controlled trial	Exposure status	Outcome event status	Low susceptibility to bias	Feasibility and generalizability constraints
Cohort	Exposure status	Outcome event status	Feasible when randomization of exposure not possible, generalizability	Susceptible to bias
Case-control	Outcome event status	Exposure status	Overcomes temporal delays and the need for huge sample sizes to accumulate rare events	Susceptible to bias

investigator identifies exposed and nonexposed groups of patients, each a cohort, and then follows them forward in time, monitoring the occurrence of the predicted outcome. The cohort design is similar to an RCT but without randomization; rather, the determination of whether a patient received the exposure of interest results from the patient or physician's preference or from happenstance.

Case-control studies also assess associations between exposures and outcomes. Rare outcomes or those that take a long time to develop can threaten the feasibility of cohort studies. The case-control study provides an alternative design that relies on the initial identification of cases—that is, patients who have already developed the target outcome—and the selection of controls—persons who do not have the outcome of interest. Using case-control designs, investigators assess the relative frequency of previous exposure to the putative harmful agent in the cases and the controls.

In a Cohort Study, Aside From the Exposure of Interest, Did the Exposed and Control Groups Start and Finish With the Same Risk for the Outcome?

Were Patients Similar for Prognostic Factors That Are Known to Be Associated With the Outcome (or Did Statistical Adjustment Level the Playing Field)?

In a cohort study, the investigator identifies exposed and nonexposed groups of patients, each a cohort, and then traces their outcomes forward in time. Cohort studies may be either prospective or retrospective. In prospective studies, the investigator starts the follow-up and waits for the outcome (events of interest) to occur. Such studies may take many years to complete and thus they are difficult to conduct. On the other hand, an advantage is that the investigator may have a better idea of how patients are to be monitored and data are to be collected. In retrospective studies, the outcomes (events of interest) have already happened at some point in the past; the investigator simply goes back even farther in the past and selects exposed and unexposed people; then the question is whether these differ in the development of these outcomes of interest. These studies are easier to perform because they depend on the availability of data on exposures and outcomes that have already happened. On the other hand, the investigator has less control over the quality and relevance of the available data for the research question being addressed.

Cohort studies of potentially harmful exposures will yield biased results if the group exposed to the putative harmful agent and the unexposed group begin with different baseline characteristics that give them a different prognosis (and the analysis fails to deal with this imbalance). Investigators rely on cohort designs when exposure has little or no possible benefit and possible harm (making randomization unethical) or when harmful outcomes occur infrequently.

In an example of the latter situation, clinically apparent upper gastrointestinal hemorrhage in nonsteroidal anti-inflammatory drug (NSAID) users occurs approximately 1.5 times per 1000 person-years of exposure, in comparison with 1.0 per 1000 person-years in those not taking NSAIDs.[10] Because the event rate in unexposed patients is so low (0.1%), an RCT to study an increase in risk of 50% would require huge numbers of patients (sample size calculations suggest about 75 000 patients per group) for adequate power to test the hypothesis that NSAIDs cause the additional bleeding.[11] Such an RCT would not be feasible, but a cohort study, in which the information comes from a large administrative database, would be possible.

One danger in using observational studies to assess a possible harmful exposure is that exposed and unexposed patients may begin with a different risk of the target outcome. For instance, in the association between NSAIDs and the increased risk of upper gastrointestinal bleeding, age may be associated with both exposure to NSAIDs and gastrointestinal bleeding. In other words, because patients taking NSAIDs will be older and because older patients are more likely to bleed, this confounding variable makes attribution of an increased risk of bleeding to NSAID exposure problematic.

There is no reason that patients who self-select (or who are selected by their physician) for exposure to a potentially harmful agent should be similar to the nonexposed patients with respect to other important determinants of that outcome. Indeed, there are many reasons to expect they will not be similar. Physicians are reluctant to prescribe medications they perceive will put their patients at risk and can selectively prescribe low-risk medications.

In one study, for instance, 24.1% of patients who were given a then-new NSAID, ketoprofen, had received peptic ulcer therapy during the previous 2 years in comparison with 15.7% of the control population.[12] The likely reason is that the ketoprofen manufacturer succeeded in persuading clinicians that ketoprofen was less likely to cause gastrointestinal bleeding than other agents. A comparison of ketoprofen to other agents would be subject to the risk of finding a spurious increase in bleeding with the new agent (compared with other therapies) because higher-risk patients would have been receiving the ketoprofen.

The prescription of benzodiazepines to elderly patients provides another example of the way that selective physician prescribing practices can lead to a different distribution of risk in patients receiving particular medications, sometimes hundreds of thousands of participants. By contrast, using the case-control strategy, the investigators delineated 2 relatively small groups of young women. Those who had the outcome of interest (vaginal adenocarcinoma) were designated as the cases ($n = 8$) and those who did not experience the outcome were designated as the controls ($n = 32$). Then working backward in time, they determined exposure rates to DES for the 2 groups. The investigators found a strong association between in utero DES exposure and vaginal adenocarcinoma, which was extremely unlikely to be attributable to the play of chance ($P < .001$) They found their answer without a delay of 20 years and by studying only 40 women.

A critical issue in that study would be whether the cases would have had any other special circumstances to be exposed to DES that controls would not. In this situation, DES had been prescribed to woman at risk for miscarriages or having premature births. It would be important in the assessment of this study to be confident that those risk factors on their own could not account for the subsequent high rate of vaginal pathology in the female offspring.

In another study, investigators used a case-control design relying on computer record linkages between health insurance data and a drug plan to investigate the possible relationship between use of β-adrenergic agonists and mortality rates in patients with asthma.[20] The database for the study included 95% of the population of the province of Saskatchewan in western Canada. The investigators used matching to choose 129 cases of fatal or near-fatal asthma attack with 655 controls that also had asthma but who had not had a fatal or near-fatal asthma attack.

The tendency of patients with more severe asthma to use more β-adrenergic medications could create a spurious association between drug use and mortality rate. The investigators attempted to control for the confounding effect of disease severity by measuring the number of hospitalizations in the 24 months before death (for the cases) or before the index

referred to as the channeling bias.[13] Ray et al[14] found an association between long-acting benzodiazepines and risk of falls (relative risk [RR], 2.0; 95% confidence interval [CI], 1.6-2.5) in data from 1977 to 1979 but not in data from 1984 to1985 (RR, 1.3; 95% CI, 0.9-1.8). The most plausible explanation for the change is that patients at high risk for falls (those with dementia) selectively received these benzodiazepines during the earlier period. Reports of associations between benzodiazepine use and falls led to greater caution, and the apparent association disappeared when physicians began to avoid using benzodiazepines in those at high risk of falling.

Therefore, investigators must document the characteristics of the exposed and nonexposed participants and either demonstrate their comparability or use statistical techniques to create a level playing field by adjusting for differences. Effective adjusted analyses for prognostic factors require the accurate measurement of those prognostic factors. For prospective cohorts, the investigators may take particular care of the quality of this information. For retrospective databases, however, one has to make use of what is available. Large administrative databases, although providing a sample size that allows ascertainment of rare events, sometimes have limited quality of data concerning relevant patient characteristics.

For example, Jollis et al[15] wondered about the accuracy of information about patient characteristics in an insurance claims database. To investigate this issue, they compared the insurance claims data with prospective data collection by a cardiology fellow. They found a high degree of chance-corrected agreement between the fellow and the administrative database for the presence of diabetes: the κ, a measure of chance-corrected agreement, was 0.83. They also found a high degree of agreement for myocardial infarction (κ, 0.76) and moderate agreement for hypertension (κ, 0.56). However, agreement was poor for heart failure (κ, 0.39) and very poor for tobacco use (κ, 0.19)

Even if investigators document the comparability of potentially confounding variables in exposed and nonexposed cohorts and even if they use statistical techniques to adjust for differences, important prognostic factors that the investigators do not know about or have not measured may be unbalanced between the groups and thus may be responsible for differences in outcome. We call this residual confounding. Returning to our earlier example, for instance, it may be that the illnesses that require NSAIDs, rather than the NSAIDs themselves, can contribute to the increased risk of bleeding. Thus, the strength of inference from a cohort study will always be less than that of a rigorously conducted RCT.

Were the Circumstances and Methods for Detecting the Outcome Similar?

In RCTs and cohort studies, ascertainment of outcome is the key issue. For example, investigators have reported a 3-fold increase in the risk of malignant melanoma in individuals working with radioactive materials. One possible explanation for some of the increased risk might be that physicians, concerned about a possible risk, search more diligently and therefore detect disease that might otherwise go unnoticed (or they may detect disease at an earlier point in time). This could result in the exposed cohort having an apparent, but spurious, increase in risk—a situation we refer to as surveillance bias.[16]

The choice of outcome may partially address this problem. In one cohort study, for example, investigators assessed perinatal outcomes among infants of men exposed to lead and organic solvents in the printing industry by means of a cohort study assessing all the men who had been members of the printers' unions in Oslo.[17] The investigators used job classification to categorize the fathers as either being exposed to lead and organic solvents or not exposed to those substances. Investigators' awareness of whether the fathers had been exposed to the lead or solvents might bias their assessment of the baby's outcome for minor birth defects or for defects that required special investigative procedures. On the other hand, the outcome of preterm birth would be less susceptible to a detection bias. In the study,

exposure was associated with an 8-fold increase in preterm births, but it was not linked with birth defects, so detection bias was unlikely.

Was the Follow-up Sufficiently Complete?

As we pointed out in Chapter 6, Therapy, loss to follow-up can introduce bias because the patients who are lost may have different outcomes from those patients still available for assessment. This is particularly problematic if there are differences in follow-up between the exposed and nonexposed groups.

In a well-executed study,[18] investigators determined the vital status of 1235 of 1261 white men (98%) employed in a chrysotile asbestos textile operation between 1940 and 1975. The RR for lung cancer death over time increased from 1.4 to 18.2 in direct proportion to the cumulative exposure among asbestos workers with at least 15 years since first exposure. In this study, where exposure was on a continuum (ie, not dichotomous), the 2% missing data were unlikely to affect the results, and the loss to follow-up did not threaten the validity of the inference that asbestos exposure caused lung cancer deaths.

In a Case-Control Study, Did the Cases and Control Group Have the Same Risk (Chance) for Being Exposed in the Past?

Were Cases and Controls Similar With Respect to the Indication or Circumstances That Would Lead to Exposure?

Investigators used a case-control design to demonstrate the association between diethylstilbestrol (DES) ingestion by pregnant women and the development of vaginal adenocarcinomas in their daughters many years later.[19] An RCT or prospective cohort study designed to test this cause-and-effect relationship would have required at least 20 years from the time when the association was first suspected until the completion of the study. Further, given the infrequency of the disease, either an RCT or a cohort study would have required

date of entry into the study (for the control group) and by using an index of the aggregate use of medications. They found an association between the routine use of large doses of β-adrenergic agonist-metered dose inhalers and death from asthma (odds ratio [OR], 2.6 per canister per month; 95% CI, 1.7-3.9), even after correcting for their measures of disease severity.

As with cohort studies, case-control studies are susceptible to unmeasured confounding variables, particularly when exposure varies over time. For instance, previous hospitalization and medication use may not adequately capture all the variability in underlying disease severity in asthma. In addition, adverse lifestyle behaviors of asthmatic patients who use large amounts of β-agonists could be the real explanation for the association.

Were the Circumstances and Methods for Determining Exposure Similar for Cases and Controls?

In case-control studies, ascertainment of the exposure is a key issue. If case patients have a better memory for exposure than control patients, the result will be a spurious association.

For example, a case-control study found a 2-fold increase in risk of hip fracture associated with psychotropic drug use. In this study, investigators established drug exposure by examining computerized claims files of the Michigan Medicaid program, a strategy that avoided selective memory of exposure—recall bias—and differential probing of cases and controls by an interviewer—interviewer bias.[21]

Another example is a study that evaluated whether the use of cellular phones increases the risk of motor vehicle crash. Suppose the investigators had tried to ask people who had a motor vehicle crash and control patients (who were in no crash at the same day and time) whether they were using their cellular phone around the time of interest. People who were in a crash would have been more likely to recall such use because their memory might be heightened by the unfortunate circumstances. This would have led to a spurious relationship because of differential recall. Therefore, the investigators in this study instead used a computerized database of cellular phone use. Moreover, they used each person in a crash as his or her own control: the time of the crash was matched against corresponding times of the life of the same person when they were driving but when no crash occurred (eg, same time driving to work). This appropriate design established that use of cellular phones increases the risk of having a motor vehicle crash.[22]

Not all studies have access to unbiased information on exposure. In a case-control study looking at the association between coffee and pancreatic cancer, the patients with cancer may be more motivated to identify possible explanations for their problem and provide a greater recounting of coffee use.[23] Also, if the interviewers are not blinded to whether a patient is a case or a control patient, the interviewer may probe deeper for exposure information from cases. In this particular study, there were no objective sources of data regarding exposure. Recall or interviewer bias may explain the apparent association.

As it turns out, another bias provides an even more likely explanation for what turned out to be a spurious association. The investigators chose control patients from the practices of the physicians looking after the patients with pancreatic cancer. These control patients had a variety of gastrointestinal problems, some of which were exacerbated by coffee ingestion. The control patients had learned to avoid coffee, which explains the investigators' finding of an association between coffee (which the pancreatic cancer patients consumed at general population levels) and pancreatic cancer. Subsequent investigations, using more appropriate controls, refuted the association.[24]

The examples above relate to the biased assessment of exposure, but the inaccurate assessment of exposure may also be random. In other words, lots of exposed persons get classified as unexposed, and vice versa, but the rates of misclassification are similar in cases and controls. Such nondifferential misclassification tends to dilute the association (ie, the true association will be larger than the observed association). In the extreme case in which errors are very frequent, even associations that are very strong in reality may not be identified in the database.

Cross-Sectional Studies

Like the cohort and the case-control study, the cross-sectional study is also an observational study design. Like a cohort study, a cross-sectional study is based on an assembled population of exposed and unexposed subjects. But in the cross-sectional study, the exposure and the existing or prevalent outcome are measured at the same time. Accordingly, the direction of association may be difficult to determine. Another important limitation is that the outcome, or the threat of getting it, may have led to a departure of cases, so that a measure of association may be biased against the association. However, cross-sectional studies are relatively inexpensive and quick to conduct and may be useful in generating and exploring hypotheses that will be subsequently investigated using other observational designs or RCTs.

Case Series and Case Reports

Case series (descriptions of a series of patients) and case reports (descriptions of individual patients) do not provide any comparison group, so it is impossible to determine whether the observed outcome would likely have occurred in the absence of the exposure. Although descriptive studies occasionally demonstrate dramatic findings mandating an immediate change in physician behavior as a precaution, before the availability of evidence from stronger study designs (eg, recall the consequences of case reports of specific birth defects occurring in association with thalidomide exposure),[25] there are potentially undesirable consequences when actions are taken in response to weak evidence.

Consider the case of the drug Bendectin (a combination of doxylamine, pyridoxine, and dicyclomine used as an antiemetic in pregnancy), whose manufacturer withdrew it from the market as a consequence of case reports suggesting that it was teratogenic.[26] Later, although a number of comparative studies demonstrated the drug's relative safety,[27] they could not eradicate the prevailing litigious atmosphere—which prevented the manufacturer from reintroducing Bendectin. Thus, many pregnant women who might have benefited from the drug's availability were denied the symptomatic relief it could have offered.

For some interventions, registries of adverse events may provide the best possible evidence initially. For example, there are vaccine registries that record adverse events among people who have received the vaccine. These registries may signal problems with a particular adverse event that would be very difficult to capture from prospective studies (too small sample size). Even retrospective studies might be too difficult to conduct if most people receive the vaccine or the people who do not receive the vaccine may be quite different from those who get it, and the differences cannot be accounted for adequately. In this case, a before/after comparison using the general population before the introduction of the new vaccine can be conducted. But such comparisons using historical controls are prone to bias because many other things may have changed in the same period. However, if changes in the incidence of an adverse event are very large, the signal may be real. An example is the clustering of intussusception cases among children receiving rotavirus vaccine,[28] resulting in a decision to withdraw the vaccine. The association was subsequently strengthened by a case-control study.[29]

In general, clinicians should not draw conclusions about cause-and-effect relationships from case series, but rather, they should recognize that the results may generate questions for regulatory agencies, which clinical investigators should address with valid studies. When the immediate risk of exposure outweighs the benefits (and outweighs the risk of stopping an exposure), the clinician may have to make a management decision with less than optimal data.

Design Issues: Summary

Just as it is true for the resolution of questions of therapeutic effectiveness, clinicians should first look to RCTs to resolve issues of harm. They will often be disappointed in the search and must make use of studies of weaker design. Regardless of the design, however, they should look for an appropriate control population before making a strong inference about a putative harmful agent. For RCTs and cohort studies, the control group should have a similar baseline risk of outcome, or investigators should use statistical techniques to adjust or correct for differences. In case-control studies, the cases and the controls should have had a similar opportunity to have been exposed, so that if a difference in exposure is observed one might legitimately conclude that the association could be due to a causal link between the exposure and the outcome and not due to a confounding factor. Alternatively, investigators should use statistical techniques to adjust for differences.

Even when investigators have taken all the appropriate steps to minimize bias, clinicians should bear in mind that residual differences between groups may still bias the results of observational studies.[30] Because evidence, provider preferences, and patient values and preferences determine the use of interventions in the real world, exposed and unexposed patients are likely to differ in prognostic factors.

The extent of bias in observational studies vs randomized trials remains uncertain. An empirical evaluation of 15 harms in which both types of evidence were available showed that observational studies might give either smaller or larger risk estimates compared with RCTs, but it is more common for observational studies to underestimate rather than overestimate the absolute risk of harm.[31] Therefore, evidence of harmful effects from well-designed observational studies should not be easily dismissed.

USING THE GUIDE

Returning to our earlier discussion, the study that we retrieved investigating the association between soy milk (or formula) and the development of peanut allergy used a case-control design.[1] Those with peanut allergy (cases) appear to be similar to the controls with respect to the indication or circumstances leading to soy exposure, but there were a few potentially important imbalances. In the peanut allergy group (cases), both a family history of peanut allergy and an older sibling with a history of milk intolerance were more common and could bias the likelihood of a subsequent child's being exposed to soy. To avoid confounding, these factors were adjusted in the analysis to provide an independent assessment of the association between soy and peanut allergy.

The methods for determining exposure were similar for cases and controls because the data were collected prospectively and both the interviewers and parents were unaware of the hypothesis relating soy exposure to peanut allergy (thus avoiding interviewer and perhaps recall bias). With regard to access to soy, all the children came from the same geographic region, although this does not ensure that cultural and economic factors that might determine soy access were balanced between cases and controls. Thus, from the initial assessment, the validity of the study appears adequate with the appropriate adjustments being done.

WHAT ARE THE RESULTS?

How Strong Is the Association Between Exposure and Outcome?

We describe the alternatives for expressing the association between the exposure and the outcome—the RR and the OR—in other chapters of this book (see Chapter 6, Therapy, and Chapter 7, Does Treatment Lower Risk? Understanding the Results).

In a cohort study assessing in-hospital mortality after noncardiac surgery in male veterans, 23 of 289 patients with a history of hypertension died compared with 3 of 185 patients without the condition. The RR for mortality in hypertensive patients[32] (23/289 and 3/185) was 4.9. The RR tells us that death after noncardiac surgery occurs almost 5 times more often in patients with hypertension than in normotensive patients.

The estimate of RR depends on the availability of samples of exposed and unexposed patients, where the proportion of the patients with the outcome of interest can be determined. The RR is therefore not applicable to case-control studies in which the number of cases and controls—and, therefore, the proportion of individuals with the outcome—is chosen by the investigator. For case-control studies, instead of using a ratio of RR, we use OR, the odds of a case patient being exposed divided by the odds of a control patient being exposed (see Chapter 7, Does Treatment Lower Risk; Understanding the Results). In circumstances in which the outcome is rare in the population at large (< 1%), the OR of a case-control study represents the risk ratio in the whole population from which the cases and controls have been sampled. Even when event rates are as high as 10%, the OR and RR may still be quite close.

When considering both study design and strength of association, we may be ready to interpret a small increase in risk as representing a true harmful effect if the study design is strong (such as in an RCT). A much greater increase in risk might be required of weaker designs (such as cohort or case-control studies) because subtle findings are more likely to be caused by the inevitably higher chance of bias. Very large values of RR or OR represent strong associations that are less likely to be the result of bias.

In addition to showing a large magnitude of RR or OR, there is a second finding that can strengthen an inference that an exposure is truly associated with harmful effect. If, when the quantity or the duration of exposure to the putative harmful agent increases, the risk for the adverse outcome also increases (ie, the data suggest a dose-response gradient), then we are more likely to be dealing with a causal relationship between exposure and outcome. The fact that the risk of dying from lung cancer in male physician smokers increases by 50%, 132%, and 220% for 1 to 14, 15 to 24, and 25 or more cigarettes smoked per day, respectively, strengthens our inference that cigarette smoking causes lung cancer.[33]

How Precise Is the Estimate of the Risk?

Clinicians can evaluate the precision of the estimate of risk by examining the CI around that estimate (see Chapter 6, Therapy; see also Chapter 8, Confidence Intervals). In a study in which investigators have shown an association between an exposure and an adverse outcome, the lower limit of the estimate of RR associated with the adverse exposure provides an estimate of the lowest possible magnitude of the association. Alternatively, in a negative study (in which the results are not statistically significant) the upper boundary of the CI around the RR tells the clinician just how big an adverse effect may still be present, despite the failure to show a statistically significant association (see Chapter 8, Confidence Intervals).

USING THE GUIDE

The investigators calculated the OR for the risk of peanut allergy in those exposed to soy vs those not exposed to be 2.6 (95% CI, 1.3-5.2). These results were adjusted for skin manifestations of allergy (ie, atopy). The consumption of soy by the infants was independently associated with peanut allergy and could not be explained as a dietary response to other atopic conditions. It nevertheless remains possible that the association with soy was confounded by other, unknown factors.[1] Unfortunately, the investigators did not address the possibility of a dose-response relationship for soy exposure and the development of peanut allergy.

HOW CAN I APPLY THE RESULTS TO PATIENT CARE?

Were the Study Patients Similar to the Patient in My Practice?

If possible biases in a study are not sufficient to dismiss the study out of hand, you should consider the extent to which the results might apply to the patient in your practice. Could your patient have met the eligibility criteria? Is your patient similar to those described in the study with respect to potentially important factors, such as patient characteristics or medical history? If not, is the biology of the harmful exposure likely to be different for the patient for whom you are providing care?

Was Follow-up Sufficiently Long?

Studies can be pristine in terms of validity but of limited use if patients are not followed up for a sufficiently long period. That is, they may provide an unbiased estimate of the effect of an exposure during the short term, but the effect we are really interested in is during a longer period. For example, most cancers take a decade or longer to develop from the original assault at the biologic level to the clinically detected malignancy. For example, if the question is whether a specific exposure, say to an industrial chemical, causes cancer to develop, one would not expect cancers detected in the first few years to reflect any of the effect of the exposure under question.

Is the Exposure Similar to What Might Occur in My Patient?
Are There Important Differences in the Exposures, for Instance, Dose or Duration, Between Your Patients and the Patients in the Study?

As an illustration, the risk of thrombophlebitis associated with oral contraceptive use described in the 1970s may not be applicable to the patient in the 21st century because of the lower estrogen dose in oral contraceptives currently used. Another example comes from the study that showed that workers employed in chrysotile asbestos textile operation between 1940 and 1975 had an increased risk for lung cancer death, a risk that increased from 1.4 to 18.2 in direct relation to cumulative exposure among asbestos workers with at least 15 years since first exposure.[18] The study does not provide reliable information regarding what might be the risks associated with only brief or intermittent exposure to asbestos (eg, a person working for a few months in an office located in a building subsequently found to have abnormally high asbestos levels).

What Is the Magnitude of the Risk?
The RR and OR do not tell us how frequently the problem occurs; they tell us only that the observed effect occurs more or less often in the exposed group compared with the unexposed group. Thus, we need a method for assessing clinical importance. In our discussion of therapy (see Chapter 6, Therapy; and Chapter 7, Does Treatment Lower Risk? Understanding the Results), we described how to calculate the number of patients whom clinicians must treat to prevent an adverse event

(number needed to treat). When the issue is harm, we can use data from a randomized trial or cohort study in a similar way, only this time to calculate the number of patients that would have to be exposed to result in 1 additional harmful event. We may even use data from case-control studies with OR, although the formula is a bit more complex, and we would need to know the event rate for the outcome in the unexposed population from which the cases and controls were drawn.

During an average of 10 months of follow-up, investigators conducting the Cardiac Arrhythmia Suppression Trial, an RCT of antiarrhythmic agents,[34] found that the mortality rate at approximately 10 months was 3.0% for placebo-treated patients and 7.7% for those treated with either encainide or flecainide. The absolute risk increase was 4.7%, the reciprocal of which tells us that, on average, for every 21 patients treated with encainide or flecainide for about a year, we would cause 1 excess death. This contrasts with our example of the association between NSAIDs and upper gastrointestinal bleeding. Of 2000 unexposed patients, 2 will have a bleeding episode each year. Of 2000 patients taking NSAIDs, 3 will have such an episode each year. Thus, if we treat 2000 patients with NSAIDs, we can expect a single additional bleeding event.[10]

Are There Any Benefits That Offset the Risks Associated With Exposure?

Even after evaluating the evidence that an exposure is harmful and establishing that the results are potentially applicable to the patient in your practice, determining subsequent actions may not be simple. In addition to considering the magnitude of the risk, one must consider what are the adverse consequences of reducing or eliminating exposure to the harmful agent; that is, the magnitude of any potential benefit that patients will no longer receive.

Clinical decision making is simple when harmful consequences are unacceptable and benefit is absent. Because the evidence of increased mortality from encainide and flecainide came from an RCT, we can be confident of the causal connection. Because treating only 21 people would result in an excess death, it is no wonder that clinicians quickly curtailed their use of these antiarrhythmic agents when the study results became available.

The clinical decision is also made easier when an acceptable alternative for avoiding the risk is available. Even if the evidence is relatively weak, the availability of an alternative substance can result in a clear decision.

> For instance, the early case-control studies demonstrating the association between aspirin use and Reye syndrome were relatively weak and left considerable doubt about the causal relationship. Although the strength of the inference was not great, the availability of a safe, inexpensive, and well-tolerated alternative, acetaminophen, justified the preference for using this alternative agent in lieu of aspirin in children at risk for Reye syndrome.[35]
>
> In contrast to the early studies regarding aspirin and Reye syndrome, multiple well-designed cohort and case-control studies have consistently demonstrated an association between NSAIDs and upper gastrointestinal bleeding; therefore, our inference about harm has been relatively strong. However, the risk of an upper gastrointestinal bleeding episode is quite low, and there may not be safer and equally efficacious anti-inflammatory alternatives available. We were therefore probably right in continuing to prescribe NSAIDs for the appropriate clinical conditions.

USING THE GUIDE

You determine that the patient's unborn child, once he or she reaches early childhood, would likely fulfill the eligibility criteria in the study. Also relevant to the clinical scenario, but perhaps unknown, is whether the soy products discussed in the study are similar to the ones that the patient is considering using. With regard to the magnitude of risk, we are told that the prevalence of peanut allergy is approximately 4 per 1000 children. An approximate calculation would suggest that with exposure to soy, 10 children per 1000 would be affected by peanut allergy. In other words, the number of children needed to be exposed to soy that would result in 1 additional case of peanut allergy is 167. (This estimate is crude and relies on a number of unverified assumptions regarding the true incidence of peanut allergy.) Finally, there are no data regarding the negative consequences of withholding soy formula or soy milk products, and this would clearly be dependent on how severe and sustained an intolerance to cow's milk was in a particular child.

CLINICAL RESOLUTION

To decide on your course of action, you proceed through the 3 steps of using the medical literature to guide your clinical practice. First, you consider the validity of the study before you. Adjustments of known confounders did not diminish the association between soy exposure as a neonate and the development of peanuts allergy. Also, the design of the study does not have any obvious problems with either recall or interviewer bias. Although you remain uncertain about unknown confounders, the study provides evidence of an association that one cannot easily dismiss.

Turning to the results, you note only a moderate association between soy exposure and the development of peanut allergy (2 < OR < 5). Although the results are statistically significant (ie, the 95% CI excludes 1), hidden biases and confounding could account for some or most of the magnitude of the observed OR.

You therefore proceed to the third step, with some reservations, and consider the implications of the study results for your patient. The study would appear to apply to a future child of your patient. Although the magnitude of the overall risk is small, perhaps about 1%, the consequences of peanut allergy can be a serious health threat to a patient and quite disruptive for a family because of the required precautions and food restrictions. Because the consequence of not using soy products may have minimal negative consequence and there appears to be some potential risk for increasing the likelihood of developing a peanut allergy in an infant exposed to soy, you may recommend to the mother not to use soy products unless the child is demonstrably intolerant to breast or cow's milk.

References

1. Lack G, Fox D, Northstone K, Golding J. Factors associated with the development of peanut allergy in childhood. *N Engl J Med*. 2003;348(11):977-985.

2. Lacchetti C, Ioannidis J, Guyatt G. Surprising results of randomized trials. Chapter 9.2. In: Guyatt G, Rennie D, eds. *Users' Guides to the Medical Literature: A Manual for Evidence-Based Clinical Practice*, 2nd ed. New York, NY: McGraw-Hill, 2008;113-151.

3. CAPRIE Steering Committee. A randomised, blinded, trial of clopidogrel versus aspirin in patients at risk of ischaemic events (CAPRIE). *Lancet*. 1996;348(9038):1329-1339.

4. Bennett CL, Connors JM, Carwile JM, et al. Thrombotic thrombocytopenic purpura associated with clopidogrel. *N Engl J Med*. 2000;342(24):1773-1777.

5. Silverstein FE, Graham DY, Senior JR, et al. Misoprostol reduces serious gastrointestinal complications in patients with rheumatoid arthritis receiving nonsteroidal anti-inflammatory drugs: a randomized, double-blind, placebo-controlled trial. *Ann Intern Med*. 1995;123(4):241-249.

6. Bombardier C, Laine L, Reicin A, et al; VIGOR Study Group. Comparison of upper gastrointestinal toxicity of rofecoxib and naproxen in patients with rheumatoid arthritis. *N Engl J Med*. 2000;343(21):1520-1528.

7. Langman MJ, Jensen DM, Watson DJ, et al. Adverse upper gastrointestinal effects of rofecoxib compared with NSAIDs. *JAMA*. 1999;282(20):1929-1933.

8. Papanikolaou PN, Ioannidis JP. Availability of large-scale evidence on specific harms from systematic reviews of randomized trials. *Am J Med*. 2004;117(8):582-589.

9. Ioannidis JP, Haidich AB, Pappa M, et al. Comparison of evidence of treatment effects in randomized and nonrandomized studies. *JAMA*. 2001;286(7):821-830.

10. Carson JL, Strom BL, Soper KA, West SL, Morse ML. The association of nonsteroidal anti-inflammatory drugs with upper gastrointestinal tract bleeding. *Arch Intern Med*. 1987;147(1):85-88.

11. Walter SD. Determination of significant relative risks and optimal sampling procedures in prospective and retrospective comparative studies of various sizes. *Am J Epidemiol*. 1977;105(4):387-397.

12. Leufkens HG, Urquhart J, Stricker BH, Bakker A, Petri H. Channelling of controlled release formulation of ketoprofen (Oscorel) in patients with history of gastrointestinal problems. *J Epidemiol Community Health*. 1992;46(4):428-432.

13. Joseph KS. The evolution of clinical practice and time trends in drug effects. *J Clin Epidemiol*. 1994;47(6):593-598.

14. Ray WA, Griffin MR, Downey W. Benzodiazepines of long and short elimination half-life and the risk of hip fracture. *JAMA*. 1989;262(23):3303-3307.

15. Jollis JG, Ancukiewicz M, DeLong ER, Pryor DB, Muhlbaier LH, Mark DB. Discordance of databases designed for claims payment versus clinical

information systems: implications for outcomes research. *Ann Intern Med*. 1993;119(8):844-850.

16. Hiatt RA, Fireman B. The possible effect of increased surveillance on the incidence of malignant melanoma. *Prev Med*. 1986;15(6):652-660.

17. Kristensen P, Irgens LM, Daltveit AK, Andersen A. Perinatal outcome among children of men exposed to lead and organic solvents in the printing industry. *Am J Epidemiol*. 1993;37(2):134-144.

18. Dement JM, Harris RL Jr, Symons MJ, Shy CM. Exposures and mortality among chrysotile asbestos workers, part II: mortality. *Am J Ind Med*. 1983;4(3):421-433.

19. Herbst AL, Ulfelder H, Poskanzer DC. Adenocarcinoma of the vagina: association of maternal stilbestrol therapy with tumor appearance in young women. *N Engl J Med*. 1971;284(15):878-881.

20. Spitzer WO, Suissa S, Ernst P, et al. The use of beta-agonists and the risk of death and near death from asthma. *N Engl J Med*. 1992;326(8):501-506.

21. Ray WA, Griffin MR, Schaffner W, Baugh DK, Melton LJ 3rd. Psychotropic drug use and the risk of hip fracture. *N Engl J Med*. 1987;316(7):363-369.

22. Redelmeier DA, Tibshirani RJ. Association between cellular-telephone calls and motor vehicle collisions. *N Engl J Med*. 1997;336(7):453-458.

23. MacMahon B, Yen S, Trichopoulos D, Warren K, Nardi G. Coffee and cancer of the pancreas. *N Engl J Med*. 1981;304(11):630-633.

24. Baghurst PA, McMichael AJ, Slavotinek AH, Baghurst KI, Boyle P, Walker AM. A case-control study of diet and cancer of the pancreas. *Am J Epidemiol*. 1991;134(2):167-179.

25. Lenz W. Epidemiology of congenital malformations. *Ann N Y Acad Sci*. 1965 Mar 12;123:228-236.

26. Soverchia G, Perri PF. 2 Cases of malformations of a limb in infants of mothers treated with an antiemetic in a very early phase of pregnancy. *Pediatr Med Chir*. 1981;3(1):97-99.

27. Holmes LB. Teratogen update: Bendectin. *Teratology*. 1983;27(2):277-281.

28. Centers for Disease Control and Prevention. Intussusception among recipients of rotavirus vaccine—United States, 1998-1999. *Morb Mortal Wkly Rep CDC Surveill Summ*. 1999;48(27):577-581.

29. Murphy TV, Gargiullo PM, Massoudi MS, et al. Intussusception among infants given an oral rotavirus vaccine. *N Engl J Med*. 2001;344(8):564-572.

30. Kellermann AL, Rivara FP, Rushforth NB, et al. Gun ownership as a risk factor for homicide in the home. *N Engl J Med*. 1993;329(15):1084-1091.

31. Papanikolaou PN, Christidi GD, Ioannidis JP. Comparison of evidence on harms of medical interventions in randomized and nonrandomized studies. *CMAJ*. 2006;174(5):635-641.

32. Browner WS, Li J, Mangano DT. In-hospital and long-term mortality in male veterans following noncardiac surgery: the Study of Perioperative Ischemia Research Group. *JAMA*. 1992;268(2):228-232.

33. Doll R, Hill AB. Mortality in relation to smoking: ten years' observations of British doctors. *BMJ*. 1964;1(5395):1399-1410.

34. Echt DS, Liebson PR, Mitchell LB, et al. Mortality and morbidity in patients receiving encainide, flecainide, or placebo: the Cardiac Arrhythmia Suppression Trial. *N Engl J Med*. 1991;324(12):781-788.

35. Soumerai SB, Ross-Degnan D, Kahn JS. Effects of professional and media warnings about the association between aspirin use in children and Reye's syndrome. *Milbank Q*. 1992;70(1):155-182.

THE PROCESS OF DIAGNOSIS

W. Scott Richardson and Mark C. Wilson

IN THIS CHAPTER:

CLINICAL SCENARIOS

Consider the following diagnostic situations:

1. A 43-year-old woman presents with a painful cluster of vesicles grouped in the T3 dermatome of her left thorax, which you recognize as shingles from reactivation of herpes zoster.

2. A 78-year-old man returns to the office for follow-up of hypertension. He has lost 10 kg since his last visit 4 months ago. He describes reduced appetite, but otherwise, there are no localizing symptoms. You recall that his wife died a year ago and consider depression as a likely explanation, yet his age and exposure history (ie, smoking) suggest other possibilities.

TWO COMPLEMENTARY APPROACHES TO DIAGNOSIS

The probabilistic approach to clinical diagnosis that uses *evidence* from clinical research—the focus of this chapter—complements the pattern recognition that expert clinicians use as a powerful tool (see Figure 10-1).[1-8] The first case in the opening scenario illustrates how rapidly this recognition can occur.

For more challenging or less familiar circumstances in which pattern recognition fails, clinicians can use a probabilistic mode of diagnostic thinking. Here, they generate a list of potential diagnoses, estimate the probability associated with each, and conduct investigations, the results of which increase or decrease the probabilities, until they believe they have found the answer.[9-14] The second case scenario illustrates a situation in which the clinician requires this probabilistic approach for accurate diagnosis.

Applying the probabilistic mode requires knowledge of human anatomy, pathophysiology, and the taxonomy of disease.[11,12,14] Evidence from clinical research represents another form of knowledge required for optimal diagnostic reasoning.[15-17] The remainder of this chapter will describe how evidence from clinical research can facilitate the probabilistic mode of diagnosis.

FIGURE 10-1

Pattern Recognition vs Probabilistic Diagnostic Reasoning

Pattern recognition	Probabilistic diagnostic reasoning
See it and recognize disorder	Clinical assessment generates pretest probability
↓	↓
Compare posttest probability with thresholds	New information generates posttest probability
(usually pattern recognition implies probability near 100% and so above threshold)	(may be iterative)
	↓
	Compare posttest probability with thresholds

CLUSTERS OF FINDINGS DEFINE CLINICAL PROBLEMS

Using the probabilistic mode, clinicians begin with the medical interview and physical examination, which they use to identify individual findings as potential clues. For instance, in the second scenario, the clinician noted a 10-kg weight loss in 4 months that is associated with anorexia but without localizing symptoms. Experienced clinicians often group findings into meaningful clusters, summarized in brief phrases about the symptom, body location, or organ system involved, such as "involuntary weight loss with anorexia." These clusters, often termed *clinical problems*, represent the starting point for the probabilistic approach to differential diagnosis.[11,18]

CLINICIANS SELECT A SMALL LIST OF DIAGNOSTIC POSSIBILITIES

When considering a patient's differential diagnosis, clinicians must decide which disorders to pursue. If they considered all known causes to be equally likely and tested for them all simultaneously (the "possibilistic" list), unnecessary testing would result. Instead, experienced clinicians are selective, considering first those disorders that are more likely (a probabilistic list), more serious if left undiagnosed and untreated (a prognostic list), or more responsive to treatment (a pragmatic list). Wisely selecting an individual patient's prioritized differential diagnosis involves all 3 of these considerations (probabilistic, prognostic, and pragmatic).

One might label the single best explanation for the patient's problem as the leading hypothesis or working diagnosis. In the second scenario, the clinician suspected depression as the most likely cause of the patient's anorexia and weight loss. A few (usually 1-5) other diagnoses may be worth considering at the initial evaluation because of their likelihood, seriousness if undiagnosed and untreated, or responsiveness to treatment. In the case of unexplained weight loss, the man's age raises the specter of neoplasm, and in particular, his past smoking suggests the possibility of lung cancer.

Additional causes of the problem may be too unlikely to consider at the initial diagnostic evaluation but could arise subsequently if the initial hypotheses are later disproved. Most clinicians considering the 78-year-old man with weight loss would not select a disease that causes malabsorption as their initial differential diagnosis but might turn to this hypothesis if investigation ultimately excludes depression and cancer.

ESTIMATING THE PRETEST PROBABILITY FACILITATES THE DIAGNOSTIC PROCESS

Having assembled a short list of plausible target disorders to be investigated—the differential diagnosis for this patient—clinicians rank-order these conditions. The probabilistic approach to diagnosis encourages clinicians to estimate the probability of each target condition on the short list, the *pretest probability* (Figure 10-1).[18,19] The sum of the probabilities for all candidate diagnoses should equal 1.

How can the clinician estimate these pretest probabilities? One method is implicit, drawing on memories of previous cases with the same clinical problem(s) and using the frequency of disorders found in those previous patients to guide estimates of pretest probability for the current patient. Often, though, memory is imperfect and we are excessively influenced by particular vivid or recent experiences and by previous inferences, and we put insufficient weight on new evidence. Further, our experience with a given clinical problem may be limited. All these factors leave the probabilities arising from clinicians' intuition subject to *bias* and *random error*.[20-22]

A complementary approach uses evidence from research to guide pretest probability estimates. In one type of relevant research, patients with the same clinical problem undergo thorough diagnostic evaluation, yielding a set of frequencies of the underlying diagnoses made, which clinicians can use to estimate the initial pretest probability (see Chapter 11, Differential Diagnosis). A second category of relevant research generates clinical decision rules or prediction rules. Patients with a defined clinical problem undergo diagnostic evaluation, and investigators use statistical methods to identify clinical and diagnostic test features that segregate patients into subgroups with different probabilities of a target condition.

NEW INFORMATION GENERATES POSTTEST PROBABILITIES

Clinical diagnosis is a dynamic process. As new information arrives, it may increase or decrease the probability of a target condition or diagnosis. For instance, in the older man with involuntary weight loss, the presence of a recent major life event (his wife's death) raises the likelihood that depression is the cause, whereas the absence of localizing gut symptoms decreases the probability of an intestinal disorder. Likelihood ratios capture the extent to which new pieces of information revise probabilities (see Chapter 12, Diagnostic Tests).

Although intuitive estimates based on experience may, at times, serve clinicians well in interpreting test results, confidence in the extent to which a result increased or decreased probabilities requires systematic research. This research can take several forms, most notably individual *primary studies* of test accuracy (see Chapter 12, Diagnostic Tests) and *systematic reviews* of these test accuracy studies (see Chapter 14, Summarizing the Evidence). Once these research results have been appraised for validity and applicability, the discriminatory power of the findings or test results can be collected into reference resources useful for each clinical discipline.[23,24]

THE RELATION BETWEEN POSTTEST PROBABILITIES AND THRESHOLD PROBABILITIES DETERMINES CLINICAL ACTION

After the test result generates the posttest probability, one can compare this new probability to thresholds (Figure 10-2).[25-27] If the posttest probability is equal to 1, the diagnosis would be absolutely certain. Short of certainty, as the posttest probability approaches 1, the diagnosis becomes more and more likely and reaches a threshold of probability above which the clinician would recommend starting treatment for the disorder (the *treatment threshold*) (Figure 10-2). These thresholds apply

FIGURE 10-2

Test and Treatment Thresholds in the Diagnostic Process

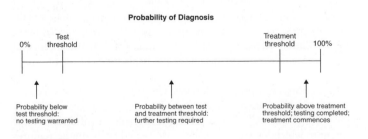

Probability of Diagnosis

0%   Test threshold   Treatment threshold   100%

Probability below test threshold: no testing warranted

Probability between test and treatment threshold: further testing required

Probability above treatment threshold; testing completed; treatment commences to both pattern recognition and probabilistic or *bayesian diagnostic reasoning* (Figure 10-1). For instance, consider the first scenario, the patient who presents with a painful eruption of grouped vesicles in the distribution of a single dermatome. In an instant, an experienced clinician would make a diagnosis of herpes zoster and consider whether to offer the patient therapy. In other words, the probability of herpes zoster is so high (near 1.0, or 100%) that it is above a threshold (the *treatment threshold*) that requires no further testing.

Alternatively, if the posttest probability equaled 0, the diagnosis would be disproved. Short of this certainty, as the posttest probability nears 0, the diagnosis becomes less and less likely, until a probability threshold is reached, below which the clinician would consider the diagnosis excluded (the test threshold).[25] Between the test and treatment thresholds are intermediate probabilities that mandate further testing. For instance, consider a previously healthy athlete who presents with lateral rib cage pain after being accidentally struck by an errant baseball pitch. Again, an experienced clinician would recognize the clinical problem (posttraumatic lateral chest pain), identify a leading hypothesis (rib contusion) and an active alternative (rib fracture), and plan a test (radiograph) to investigate the latter. If asked, the clinician could also list disorders that are too unlikely to consider further (such as myocardial infarction). In other words, although not as likely as rib contusion, the probability of a rib fracture is above a threshold for testing, whereas the probability of myocardial infarction is below the threshold for testing.

What determines these test and treatment thresholds? They are a function of the properties of the test, the disease prognosis, and the nature of the treatment. For the test threshold, the safer and less costly the testing strategy, the more serious the condition if left undiagnosed, and the more effective and safe the available treatment is, the lower we would place the test threshold. On the other hand, the less safe or more costly the test strategy, the less serious the condition if undiagnosed, and the less secure we are about the effectiveness and safety of treatment, the higher we would place the test threshold.

Consider, for instance, ordering troponin for suspected acute coronary syndrome. The condition, if present, can lead to serious consequences (such as fatal arrhythmias), and the test is inexpensive and noninvasive. This is the reason one sees emergency department physicians ordering the test for patients with even a very low probability of acute coronary syndrome; they have set a very low diagnostic threshold.

Contrast this with a pulmonary angiogram for suspected pulmonary embolism. Although the condition is serious, the test is invasive and may be complicated. As a result, if after tests such as Doppler compression ultrasonography and ventilation-perfusion scanning or helical computed tomography they are left with a low probability of pulmonary embolism, clinicians may choose to monitor closely. The test threshold is higher because of the invasiveness and risks of the test.

For the treatment threshold, the safer and the less expensive our next test, the more benign the prognosis of the illness, and the higher the costs or greater the adverse effects of the treatment options, the higher we would place the threshold, requiring greater diagnostic certainty before exposing our patients to treatment. On the other hand, the more invasive and less safe the next test needed, the more ominous the prognosis, and the safer and less costly the proposed treatment, the lower we would place the treatment threshold, as proceeding with treatment may be preferable to increasing diagnostic certainty. For instance, consider patients presenting with suspected malignancy. In general, clinicians are ready to subject such patients to invasive diagnostic tests associated with possible serious complications before treating. The reason is that the treatment—surgery, radiation, or chemotherapy—is itself associated with morbidity or even mortality. Thus, clinicians set the treatment threshold very high.

Contrast this with a patient presenting with symptoms of heartburn and acid reflux. Even if symptoms are atypical, clinicians may be ready to prescribe a proton-pump inhibitor for symptom relief rather than subject the patient to endoscopy. The lower treatment threshold is a function of the relatively benign nature of the treatment in relation to the invasiveness of the next test.

CONCLUSION

In this chapter, we outlined the probabilistic tradition of diagnostic reasoning and identified how different types of clinical research

evidence can inform our diagnostic decisions and actions. The next
chapters highlight particular aspects of the diagnostic process.

References

1. Elstein AS, Shulman L, Sprafka S. *Medical Problem Solving: An Analysis of Clinical Reasoning.* Cambridge, MA: Harvard University Press; 1978.

2. Schmidt HG, Norman GR, Boshuizen HP. A cognitive perspective on medical expertise: theory and implication. *Acad Med.* 1990;65(10):611-621.

3. Regehr G, Norman GR. Issues in cognitive psychology: implications for professional education. *Acad Med.* 1996;71(10 suppl):988-1001.

4. Redelmeier DA, Ferris LE, Tu JV, Hux JE, Schull MJ. Problems for clinical judgment: introducing cognitive psychology as one more basic science. *CMAJ.* 2001;164(3):358-360.

5. Eva KW. What every teacher needs to know about clinical reasoning. *Med Educ.* 2004;39(1):98-106.

6. Norman G. Research in clinical reasoning: past history and current trends. *Med Educ.* 2005;39(4):418-427.

7. Norman GR, Brooks LR. The non-analytical basis of clinical reasoning. *Adv Health Sci Educ.* 1997;2(2):173-184.

8. Norman GR. The epistemology of clinical reasoning: perspectives from philosophy, psychology, and neuroscience. *Acad Med.* 2000;75(10 suppl):S127-S135.

9. Barrows HS, Pickell GC. *Developing Clinical Problem Solving Skills: A Guide to More Effective Diagnosis and Treatment.* New York, NY: WW Norton; 1991.

10. Kassirer JP, Kopelman RI. *Learning Clinical Reasoning.* Baltimore, MD: Williams & Wilkins; 1991.

11. Barondess JA, Carpenter CCJ, eds. *Differential Diagnosis.* Philadelphia, PA: Lea & Febiger; 1994.

12. Bordage G. Elaborated knowledge: a key to successful diagnostic thinking. *Acad Med.* 1994;69(11):883-885.

13. Glass RD. *Diagnosis: A Brief Introduction.* Melbourne, Australia: Oxford University Press; 1996.

14. Cox K. *Doctor and Patient: Exploring Clinical Thinking.* Sydney, Australia: UNSW Press; 1999.

15. Kassirer JP. Diagnostic reasoning. *Ann Intern Med.* 1989;110(11):893-900.

16. Richardson WS. Integrating evidence into clinical diagnosis. In: Montori VM, ed. *Evidence-Based Endocrinology.* Totowa, NJ: Humana Press; 2006: 69-89.

17. Richardson WS. We should overcome the barriers to evidence-based clinical diagnosis. *J Clin Epidemiol.* 2007;60(3):217-227.

18. Richardson WS, Wilson MC, Guyatt GH, Cook DJ, Nishikawa J; Evidence-Based Medicine Working Group. Users' guides to the medical literature, XV: how to use an article about disease probability for differential diagnosis. *JAMA.* 1999;281(13):1214-1219.

19. Sox HC Jr, Blatt MA, Higgins MC, Marton KI, eds. *Medical Decision Making.* Boston, MA: Butterworth-Heinemann; 1988.

20. Richardson WS. Where do pretest probabilities come from [editorial, EBM Note]? *Evidence Based Med.* 1999;4:68-69.

21. Richardson WS, Glasziou P, Polashenski WA, Wilson MC. A new arrival—evidence about differential diagnosis [editorial]. *ACP J Club.* 2000;133(3): A11-A12.

22. Richardson WS. Five uneasy pieces about pre-test probability [editorial]. *J Gen Intern Med.* 2002;17(11):882-883.

23. Fletcher RH, Fletcher SW. *Clinical Epidemiology: The Essentials.* 4th ed. Baltimore, MD: Lippincott Williams & Wilkins; 2005.

24. Straus SE, Richardson WS, Glasziou P, Haynes RB, eds. *Evidence-Based Medicine: How to Practice and Teach EBM.* 3rd ed. Edinburgh, Scotland: Churchill-Livingstone; 2005.

25. Pauker SG, Kassirer JP. The threshold approach to clinical decision making. *N Engl J Med.* 1980;302(20):1109-1117.

26. Gross R. *Making Medical Decisions: An Approach to Clinical Decision Making for Practicing Physicians.* Philadelphia, PA: ACP Publications; 1999.

27. Hunink M, Glasziou P, eds. *Decision Making in Health and Medicine: Integrating Evidence and Values.* Cambridge, England: Cambridge University Press; 2001.

DIFFERENTIAL DIAGNOSIS

W. Scott Richardson, Mark C. Wilson,
and Thomas G. McGinn

IN THIS CHAPTER:

CLINICAL SCENARIO

A 76-Year-Old Man With Weight Loss: Which Disorders Should Be Sought and What Are Their Pretest Probabilities?

You are treating a 76-year-old man for involuntary weight loss of 10 kg in 6 months. At today's routine visit for the follow-up of his longstanding hypertension, he was surprised to be told that his weight has decreased since the last visit. He reports eating less, with little appetite but no food-related symptoms. He takes a diuretic for his hypertension, with no change in dose for more than a year, and uses acetaminophen for occasional knee pain and stiffness. He stopped smoking 11 years ago, and he stopped drinking alcohol 4 decades ago. His examination shows him to be extremely thin but provides no localizing clues. His initial blood and urine test results are normal.

You review the long list of the possible causes of involuntary weight loss, yet you realize that an exhaustive search for all possibilities at once does not appear sensible. Instead, you want more information about which causes of involuntary weight loss are common to select which disorders to pursue and to estimate the pretest probabilities for these conditions.

FINDING THE EVIDENCE

You begin by framing your knowledge gap as a question: In adults presenting with involuntary weight loss who undergo a diagnostic evaluation, how frequent are the important categories of underlying disease such as neoplasms, gastrointestinal conditions, and psychiatric disorders? As you sit in front of your computer to search for an answer, you notice your nearby files that store your article reprint collection. On a whim, you open the file for involuntary weight loss and find 1 article about the frequency of diseases in patients with involuntary weight loss that was published more than 25 years ago.[1] Hoping to find some newer evidence, you access PubMed and locate this older citation in the database. Clicking the "Related Articles" link yields 102 citations, of which the second new listing by Hernandez et al,[2] published in 2003, looks promising because it also explicitly addresses the frequency of underlying disorders in patients with weight loss.[2] Farther down the list, you find a recent narrative review article on unintentional weight loss,[3] which cites the Hernandez et al[2] article as the most recent study of causes of weight loss. To double check, you scan the chapter on weight loss in an electronic text and find that no newer study is mentioned. With some confidence that you have found the most recent evidence, you retrieve its full text to appraise critically.

Using the Guide
Table 11-1 summarizes the guides for an article about disease probabilities for differential diagnosis.

TABLE 11-1

Users' Guide for Articles About Disease Probability for Differential Diagnosis

Are the results valid?

   Did the study patients represent the full spectrum of those with this clinical problem?

   Was the diagnostic evaluation definitive?

What are the results?

   What were the diagnoses and their probabilities?

   How precise are the estimates of disease probability?

How can I apply the results to patient care?

   Are the study patients and clinical setting similar to mine?

   Is it unlikely that the disease possibilities or probabilities have changed since this evidence was gathered?

ARE THE RESULTS VALID?

Did the Study Patients Represent the Full Spectrum of Those With This Clinical Problem?

The patients in a study are drawn or sampled from an underlying target population of persons who seek care for the clinical problem being investigated. Ideally, this sample mirrors the target population in all important ways, so that the frequency of underlying diseases found in the sample reflects the frequency in the whole population. A patient sample that mirrors the target population well is termed "representative." The more representative the sample, the more accurate the resulting disease probabilities. As shown in Table 11-2, we suggest 4 ways to examine how well the study patients represent the entire target population.

First, find the investigators' definition of the presenting clinical problem because this determines the target population from which the study patients should be drawn. For instance, for a study of chest discomfort, you would want to find whether the investigators' definition included patients with chest discomfort who deny pain (like many patients with angina do), whether "chest" means discomfort only in the anterior thorax (vs also posterior), and whether patients with obvious recent trauma are excluded. In addition, investigators may specify the level of care or amount of previous evaluation, for example; "fatigue in primary care,"[4] or "referred for persistent unexplained cough."[5] Differing definitions would define differing target populations that would yield differing disease proba-

TABLE 11-2

Ensuring a Representative Patient Sample

Did the investigators define the clinical problem clearly?

Were study patients collected from all relevant clinical settings?

Were study patients recruited consecutively from the clinical settings?

Did the study patients exhibit the full clinical spectrum of this presenting problem?

bilities. A detailed, specific definition of the clinical problem allows you to recognize clearly the target population to which you will compare the patient sample assembled for the study. The less clear the definition is, the less certain you can be of the intended population, and the less confident you can be in judging how well the sample patients represent the whole and in the validity of the resulting disease probabilities.

Second, examine the settings from which patients are recruited. Patients with the same clinical problem could present to any of the different clinical settings, whether primary care offices, emergency departments, or referral clinics. The choice of where to seek care can involve several factors, including the severity of illness, the availability of various settings, the referral habits of one's clinician, or patient preferences. These influences mean that different clinical settings will treat patient groups with different disease frequencies. Typically, patients in secondary or tertiary care settings have higher proportions of more serious or less common diseases than patients treated in primary care settings. For instance, in a study of patients presenting with chest pain, a higher proportion of referral practice patients had coronary artery disease than the primary care practice patients, even among patients with similar clinical histories.[6]

Investigators should avoid restricting recruitment to idiosyncratic settings that are likely to treat an unrepresentative patient sample. For instance, for the "fatigue in primary care" problem, although only primary care settings would be relevant, the investigators would ideally recruit from a broad spectrum of primary care settings (eg, those serving patients of varying socioeconomic status). In general, the fewer the relevant sites used for patient recruitment, the greater the risk that the setting will be idiosyncratic or unrepresentative.

Third, note the investigators' methods for identifying patients at each site and how carefully they avoided missing patients. Ideally, they would recruit a consecutive sample of all patients who seek care at the study sites for the clinical problem during a specified period. If patients are not included consecutively, then unequal inclusion of patients with different underlying disorders may occur, which would reduce the representativeness of the sample and reduce confidence in the validity of the resulting disease probabilities.

Fourth, examine the spectrum of severity and clinical features exhibited by the patients in the study sample. Are mild, moderate, and severely symptomatic patients included? Are all the important variations of this presenting clinical problem found in the sample? For instance, for a study of chest discomfort, you would want to determine whether patients with chest discomfort of any degree of severity were included and whether patients were included whether they did or did not have important associated symptoms such as dyspnea, diaphoresis, or pain radiation. The fuller the clinical spectrum of patients in the sample is, the more representative the sample should be of the target population. Conversely, the narrower the clinical spectrum is, the less representative you would rate the sample and the less confidence you would have in the validity of the resulting disease probabilities.

USING THE GUIDE

Hernandez et al[2] defined the clinical problem for their study as "isolated involuntary weight loss," meaning that a verified, unintentional loss of more than 5% of body weight during 6 months occurred without localizing signs or symptoms and with no diagnosis made on initial testing. From January 1991 through December 1996, there were 1211 patients referred consecutively from a defined geographic area to their general internal medicine outpatient and inpatient settings for involuntary weight loss, of whom 306 met their definition of "isolated." Men and women are included, and ages ranged from 15 to 97 years. The sample patients' races, cultures, and socioeconomic status are not described. Patients were excluded from the sample if they lost less than 5 kg, if they had a previous diagnosis that could explain involuntary weight loss, if the initial evaluation identified the cause (eg, diuretic use in the last 3 months), or if weight loss was intentional. Thus, their study sample represents fairly well the target population of patients who are referred for the evaluation of involuntary weight loss and who are most difficult diagnostically, with only a modest restriction of the clinical spectrum.

Was the Diagnostic Evaluation Definitive?

Articles about disease probability for differential diagnosis will provide valid evidence only if the investigators arrive at correct final diagnoses for the study patients. To judge the accuracy of the final diagnoses, you should examine the diagnostic evaluation used to reach them. The more definitive this diagnostic evaluation is, the more likely it is that the frequencies of the diagnoses made in the sample are accurate estimates of the disease frequencies in the target population. As shown in Table 11-3, we suggest 6 ways to examine how definitive the diagnostic evaluation is.

First, how comprehensive is the investigators' diagnostic evaluation? Ideally, the diagnostic evaluation would be able to detect all possible causes of the clinical problem, if any are present. Within reason, the more comprehensive the set of investigations is, the smaller the chance that investigators will reach invalid conclusions about disease frequency. For example, a retrospective study of stroke in 127 patients with mental status changes failed to include a comprehensive search for all causes of delirium, and 118 cases remained unexplained.[7] Because the investigators did not describe a complete and systematic search for causes of delirium, the disease probabilities appear less credible.

Second, examine how consistently the diagnostic evaluation was carried out in the study patients. This does not mean that every patient must undergo every test. Instead, for many clinical problems, the clinician takes a detailed yet focused medical

TABLE 11-3

Ensuring a Definitive Diagnostic Evaluation

Was the diagnostic evaluation sufficiently comprehensive?

Was the diagnostic evaluation consistently applied to all patients?

Were the criteria for all candidate diagnoses explicit and credible?

Were the diagnostic labels assigned reproducibly?

Were there few patients left undiagnosed?

For undiagnosed patients, was follow-up sufficiently long and complete?

history and performs a problem-oriented physical examination of the involved organ systems, along with a few initial tests. Then, depending on the diagnostic clues from this information, further inquiry proceeds down one of multiple branching pathways. Ideally, investigators would evaluate all patients with the same initial evaluation and then follow the resulting clues using prespecified multiple branching pathways of testing. Once a definitive test result confirms a final diagnosis, further testing is unnecessary.

You may find it relatively easy to decide whether the patients' illnesses have been thoroughly and consistently investigated if they were evaluated prospectively with a predetermined diagnostic approach. When clinicians do not standardize their investigation, this becomes harder to judge. For example, in a study of precipitating factors in 101 patients with decompensated heart failure, although all patients underwent a medical history-taking and physical examination, the lack of standardization of subsequent testing makes it difficult to judge the accuracy of the disease probabilities.[8]

Third, examine the sets of criteria for each disorder used in assigning patients' final diagnoses. Ideally, investigators will develop or adapt a set of explicit criteria for each underlying candidate disorder that could be diagnosed and then apply these criteria consistently when assigning each patient a final diagnosis. When possible, these criteria should include not only the findings needed to confirm each diagnosis but also those findings useful for rejecting each diagnosis. For example, published diagnostic criteria for infective endocarditis include criteria for verifying the infection and criteria for rejecting it.[9,10] Investigators can then classify study patients into diagnostic groups that are mutually exclusive, with the exception of patients whose symptoms stem from more than 1 etiologic factor. Because a complete, explicit, referenced, and credible set of diagnostic criteria can be long, it may appear as an appendix to the printed article, such as in a study of patients with palpitations,[11] or as an electronic appendix for a Web-based publication.

While reviewing the diagnostic criteria, keep in mind that "lesion finding" is not necessarily the same thing as "illness explaining." In other words, when using credible diagnostic criteria, investigators may find that patients have 2 or more disorders that might explain the clinical problem, causing some doubt as to which disorder is the culprit. Better studies of disease probability will include some assurance that the disorders found actually did account for the patients' illnesses.

> For example, in a sequence of studies of syncope, investigators required that the symptoms occur simultaneously with an arrhythmia before that arrhythmia was judged to be the cause.[12] In a study of chronic cough, investigators gave cause-specific therapy and used positive responses to this to strengthen the case for these disorders actually causing the chronic cough.[5]

Fourth, consider whether the assignments of the patients' final diagnoses were reproducible. Ensuring reproducibility begins with the use of explicit criteria and a comprehensive and consistent evaluation, as described above. Also, investigators can use a formal test of reproducibility such as chance-corrected agreemenet (kappa), as was done in a study of causes of dizziness.[13] The greater the investigators' agreement beyond chance on the final diagnoses assigned to their patients, the more confident you can be in the validity of the resulting disease probabilities.

Fifth, look at how many patients remain undiagnosed despite the study evaluation. Ideally, a comprehensive diagnostic evaluation would leave no patient's illness unexplained, yet even the best evaluation may fall short of this goal. The higher the proportion of undiagnosed patients, the greater the chance of error in the estimates of disease probability.

> For example, in a retrospective study of various causes of dizziness in 1194 patients in an otolaryngology clinic, about 27% remained undiagnosed.[14] With more than a quarter of patients' illnesses unexplained, the disease frequencies for the overall sample might be inaccurate.

Sixth, if the study evaluation leaves some patients undiagnosed, look at the length and completeness of their follow-up and whether additional diagnoses are made and the clinical outcomes are known. The longer and more complete the follow-up, the greater our confidence in the benign nature of the conditions in patients who remain undiagnosed yet unharmed at the end of the study. How long is long enough? No single answer would satisfy all clinical problems, but we suggest 1 to

6 months for symptoms that are acute and self-limited and 1 to 5 years for chronically recurring or progressive symptoms.

USING THE GUIDE

Hernandez et al[2] described the consistent use of a standardized initial evaluation of medical history, physical examination, blood tests (blood cell counts, sedimentation rate, blood chemistries, protein electrophoresis, thyroid hormone levels), urine analysis, and radiographs (chest and abdomen), after which further testing was done at the discretion of the attending physician. The set of diagnostic criteria for each disorder is not listed. For the patients' final diagnosis, the investigators required not only finding a disorder recognized in the literature to cause weight loss but also a correlation of weight loss with the clinical outcome of the disorder (recovery or progression). Diagnostic assignments were done independently by 2 investigators, and disagreements (<5%) were resolved by consensus. An underlying disorder explaining involuntary weight loss was diagnosed for 221 (72%) patients, so 85 (28%) were initially undiagnosed. During follow-up and repeated evaluations at 3, 6, and 12 months, 55 of these 85 patients were seen, and diagnoses were made for 41, leaving 14 unexplained diagnoses at 1 year and 30 patients lost to follow-up. Thus, the reported diagnostic evaluation appears fairly credible overall, although some uncertainty exists because of unspecified criteria and the 10% loss to follow-up.

WHAT ARE THE RESULTS?

What Were the Diagnoses and Their Probabilities?

In many studies of disease probability, the authors display the main results in a table listing the diagnoses made, along with the numbers and percentages of patients found with those disorders. For some symptoms, patients may have more than 1 underlying disease coexisting with and presumably contributing to the clinical problem. In these situations, authors often identify the major diagnosis for such patients and separately tabulate contributing causes. Alternatively, authors could identify a separate multiple-etiology group.

USING THE GUIDE

Hernandez et al[2] show in a table the diagnoses made by the end of the study follow-up in 276 (90%) of their 306 patients. For instance, neoplasms were found in 104 (34%) and psychiatric diseases in 63 (21%), whereas no known cause was identified in 14 (5%).

How Precise Are the Estimates of Disease Probability?

Even when valid, these disease frequencies found in the study sample are only estimates of the true disease probabilities in the target population. You can examine the precision of these estimates with the *confidence intervals* (*CIs*) presented by the authors. If the authors do not provide them for you, you can calculate them yourself with the following formula:

$$95\% \, CI = P \pm 1.96 \times \sqrt{(P(1-P))/N}$$

where P is the proportion of patients with the etiology of interest and N is the number of patients in the sample. This formula becomes inaccurate when the number of cases is 5 or fewer, and approximations are available for this situation. For instance, consider the category of psychiatric causes of involuntary weight loss in the Hernandez et al[2] study. Using the above formula, we would start with $P = 0.23$, $(1 - P) = 0.77$, and $N = 276$. Working through the arithmetic, we find the CI to be 0.23 ± 0.049. Thus, although the measured proportion is 23%, it may range between 18.1% and 27.9%.

Whether you will deem the CIs sufficiently precise depends on where the estimated proportion and CIs fall in relation to your *test* or *treatment thresholds*. If both the estimated proportion and the entire 95% CI are on the same side of your threshold, then the result is precise enough to permit firm conclusions about disease probability for use in planning tests or treatments. Conversely, if the confidence limit around the estimate crosses your threshold, the result may not be precise enough for definitive conclusions about disease probability. A valid but imprecise probability result might still be used, keeping in mind the uncertainty and what it might mean for testing or treatment.

USING THE GUIDE

Hernandez et al[2] do not provide the 95% CIs for the probabilities they found. As we illustrate, if you were concerned about how close the probabilities were to your thresholds, you could calculate the 95% CIs yourself. In this situation, even the lower boundary of the CI appears high enough for you to pursue an underlying psychiatric disease as the cause of involuntary weight loss.

HOW CAN I APPLY THE RESULTS TO PATIENT CARE?

Are the Study Patients and Clinical Setting Similar to Mine?

Earlier, we urged you to examine how the study patient sample was selected from the target population to judge the sample's representativeness and thus the validity of the results. You should now reexamine the study sample to make a different judgment—its applicability to your patients and your practice. Try asking this question framed both ways (Are the study patients and clinical setting similar enough to mine that I can use the evidence? Or, are the patients and settings so different from mine that I should disregard the results?) and compare your answers. For instance, if patients who present with this problem in your practice come from areas in which one of the underlying disorders is endemic, the probability of that condition would be much higher than its frequency found in a study done in a nonendemic area, limiting the applicability of the study results to your practice.

USING THE GUIDE

For the 76-year-old man referred to you for evaluation of involuntary weight loss, the clinical setting described by Hernandez et al[2] appears to fit fairly well. The partial description of the sample patients sounds similar enough to this man in age and sex, so that although some uncertainty may remain, they are probably not so dissimilar that this evidence cannot be used.

Is It Unlikely That the Disease Possibilities or Probabilities Have Changed Since This Evidence Was Gathered?

As time passes, evidence about disease frequency can become obsolete. Old diseases can be controlled or, as in the case of smallpox, eliminated.[15] New diseases or new epidemics of disease can arise. Such events can so alter the list of possible diseases or their likelihood that previously valid and applicable studies may lose their relevance. For example, consider how dramatically the arrival of human immunodeficiency virus transformed the possibilities and the probabilities for clinical problems such as generalized lymphadenopathy, chronic diarrhea, and involuntary weight loss.

Similar changes can occur as the result of progress in medical science or public health. For instance, in studies of fever of unknown origin, new diagnostic technologies have substantially altered the proportions of patients who are found to have malignancy or whose fevers remain unexplained.[16-18] Treatment advances that improve survival, such as chemotherapy for childhood leukemia, can bring about shifts in disease likelihood because the treatment might cause complications such as secondary malignancy years after cure of the disease. Public health measures that control diseases such as cholera can alter the likelihood of occurrence of the remaining etiologies of the clinical problems that the prevented disease would have caused; in this example, acute diarrhea.

USING THE GUIDE

The Hernandez et al[2] study was published in 2003, and the study period was 1991 to 1997. In this instance, you know of no new developments likely to change the causes or probabilities of disease in patients with involuntary weight loss since this evidence was gathered.

CLINICAL RESOLUTION

Let us return to the 76-year-old man being evaluated for involuntary weight loss. After an initial evaluation yielded no leads, a detailed interview turns up strong clues to a depressed mood with anorexia and reduced appetite after his wife died a year ago. Your leading hypothesis becomes that major depressive disorder is causing your patient's involuntary weight loss, yet this diagnosis is not sufficiently certain to stop testing to exclude other conditions. From the Hernandez et al[2] study, you decide to include in your active alternatives selected neoplasms (common, serious, and treatable) and hyperthyroidism (less common yet serious and treatable), and you arrange testing to exclude these disorders (ie, these alternatives are above your test threshold). Finally, given that few of the study patients had a malabsorption syndrome, and because your patient has no other features of this disorder besides involuntary weight loss, you place it into your "other hypotheses" category (ie, below your test threshold) and decide to delay testing for this condition. You use the disease frequencies from the study as starting estimates for pretest probability and then raise the probability for depression, given the clues, which lowers the probabilities for the other conditions.

References

1. Marton KI, Sox HC Jr, Krupp JR. Involuntary weight loss: diagnostic and prognostic significance. *Ann Intern Med.* 1981;95(5):568-574.

2. Hernandez JL, Riancho JA, Matorras P, Gonzalez-Macias J. Clinical evaluation for cancer in patients with involuntary weight loss without specific symptoms. *Am J Med.* 2003;114(8):631-637.

3. Alibhai SMH, Greenwood C, Payette H. An approach to the management of unintentional weight loss in elderly people. *CMAJ.* 2005;172(6):773-780.

4. Elnicki DM, Shockcor WT, Brick JE, Beynon D. Evaluating the complaint of fatigue in primary care: diagnoses and outcomes. *Am J Med.* 1992;93(3):303-306.

5. Pratter MR, Bartter T, Akers S, et al. An algorithmic approach to chronic cough. *Ann Intern Med.* 1993;119(10):977-983.

6. Sox HC, Hickam DH, Marton KI, et al. Using the patient's history to estimate the probability of coronary artery disease: a comparison of primary care and referral practices. *Am J Med.* 1990;89(1):7-14.

7. Benbadis SR, Sila CA, Cristea RL. Mental status changes and stroke. *J Gen Intern Med.* 1994;9(9):485-487.

8. Ghali JK, Kadakia S, Cooper R, Ferlinz J. Precipitating factors leading to decompensation of heart failure: traits among urban blacks. *Arch Intern Med.* 1988;148(9):2013-2016.

9. von Reyn CF, Levy BS, Arbeit RD, Friedland G, Crumpacker CS. Infective endocarditis: an analysis based on strict case definitions. *Ann Intern Med.* 1981;94(4 pt 1):505-517.

10. Durack DT, Lukes AS, Bright DK; Duke Endocarditis Service. New criteria for diagnosis of infective endocarditis: utilization of specific echocardiographic findings. *Am J Med.* 1994;96(3):200-209.

11. Weber BE, Kapoor WN. Evaluation and outcomes of patients with palpitations. *Am J Med.* 1996;100:138-148.

12. Kapoor WN. Evaluation and outcome of patients with syncope. *Medicine.* 1990;69:160-175.

13. Kroenke K, Lucas CA, Rosenberg ML, et al. Causes of persistent dizziness: a prospective study of 100 patients in ambulatory care. *Ann Intern Med.* 1992;117(11):898-904.

14. Katsarkas A. Dizziness in aging—a retrospective study of 1194 cases. *Otolaryngol Head Neck Surg.* 1994;110(3):296-301.

15. Barquet N, Domingo P. Smallpox: the triumph over the most terrible of the ministers of death. *Ann Intern Med.* 1997;127(8 pt 1):635-642.

16. Petersdorf RG, Beeson PB. Fever of unexplained origin: report on 100 cases. *Medicine.* 1961;40:1-30.

17. Larson EB, Featherstone HJ, Petersdorf RG. Fever of undetermined origin: diagnosis and follow up of 105 cases, 1970-1980. *Medicine.* 1982;61 (5):269-292.

18. Knockaert DC, Vanneste LJ, Vanneste SB, Bobbaers HJ. Fever of unknown origin in the 1980s: an update of the diagnostic spectrum. *Arch Intern Med.* 1992;152(1):51-55.

DIAGNOSTIC TESTS

Toshi A. Furukawa, Sharon Strauss,
Heiner C. Bucher, and Gordon Guyatt

IN THIS CHAPTER:

Will the Test Results Change My Management Strategy?

Will Patients Be Better Off as a Result of the Test?

INTRODUCTION

In the previous 2 chapters (Chapter 10, The Process of Diagnosis, and Chapter 11, Differential Diagnosis), we explained the process of diagnosis, the way diagnostic test results move clinicians across the test threshold and the therapeutic threshold, and how to use studies to help obtain an accurate *pretest probability*. In this chapter, we show you how to use an article addressing the ability of a diagnostic test to move clinicians toward the extremely high (ruling in) and extremely low (ruling out) *posttest probabilities* they seek.

CLINICAL SCENARIO

How Can We Identify Dementia Quickly and Accurately?

You are a busy primary care practitioner with a large proportion of elderly patients in your practice. Earlier in the day, you treated a 70-year-old woman who lives alone and has been managing well. On this visit, she complained about a longstanding problem, joint pain in her lower extremities. During the visit, you have the impression that, as you put it to yourself, "she isn't quite all there," although you find it hard to specify further. On specific questioning about memory and function, she acknowledges that her memory is not what it used to be but otherwise denies problems. Pressed for time, you deal with the osteoarthritis and move on to the next patient.

That evening, you ponder the problem of making a quick assessment of your elderly patients when the possibility of cognitive impairment occurs to you. The Mini-Mental Status Examination (MMSE), with which you are familiar, takes too long. You wonder whether there are any brief instruments that allow a reasonably accurate rapid diagnosis of cognitive impairment to help you identify patients who need more extensive investigation.

FINDING THE EVIDENCE

You formulate the clinical question: In older patients with suspected cognitive impairment, what is the accuracy of a brief screening tool for diagnosing dementia (or for identifying those who need more extensive investigation)? You select "diagnosis" and "narrow, specific search" from the PubMed Clinical Queries page. Using search terms "dementia AND screen* AND brief," the search yields 48 citations. Limiting to English-language studies of human beings in the last 5 years cuts the list to 21. You survey the abstracts, looking for articles that focus on patients with suspected dementia and report accuracy similar to your previous standard, the MMSE. An article reporting results for an instrument named Six-Item Screener (SIS) meets both criteria.[1] You retrieve the full-text article electronically and start to read it, hoping its methods and results will justify using the instrument in your office.

ARE THE RESULTS VALID?

Table 12-1 summarizes our Users' Guides for assessing the validity, examining the results, and determining the applicability of a study reporting on the accuracy of a diagnostic test.

Did Participating Patients Present a Diagnostic Dilemma?

A diagnostic test is useful only if it distinguishes between conditions and disorders that might otherwise be confusing. Although most tests can differentiate healthy persons from severely affected ones, this ability will not help us in clinical practice. Studies that confine themselves to florid cases versus asymptomatic healthy volunteers are unhelpful because, when the diagnosis is obvious, we do not need a diagnostic test. Only a study that closely resembles clinical practice and includes patients with mild, early manifestations of the target condition can establish a test's true value.

TABLE 12-1

Users' Guide for an Article About Interpreting Diagnostic Test Results

Are the results valid?

- Did participating patients present a diagnostic dilemma
- Did investigators compare the test to an appropriate, independent reference standard?
- Were those interpreting the test and reference standard blind to the other results?
- Did investigators perform the same reference standard to all patients regardless of the results of the test under investigation?

What are the results?

- What likelihood ratios were associated with the range of possible test results?

How can I apply the results to patient care?

- Will the reproducibility of the test result and its interpretation be satisfactory in my clinical setting?
- Are the study results applicable to the patients in my practice?
- Will the test results change my management strategy?
- Will patients be better off as a result of the test?

The story of carcinoembryonic antigen (CEA) testing in patients with colorectal cancer shows how choosing the wrong spectrum of patients can dash the hopes raised with the introduction of a diagnostic test. A study found that CEA was elevated in 35 of 36 people with known advanced cancer of the colon or rectum. The investigators found much lower levels in normal people, pregnant women, or in patients with a variety of other conditions.[2] The results suggested that CEA might be useful in diagnosing colorectal cancer or even in screening for the disease. In subsequent studies of patients with less advanced stages of colorectal cancer (and therefore lower disease severity) and patients with other cancers or other gastrointestinal disorders (and therefore different but potentially confused disorders), the accuracy of CEA testing as a diagnostic tool plummeted. Clinicians appropriately abandoned CEA measurement for new cancer diagnosis and screening.

There have been 3 systematic, empirical examinations of design-related *bias* in studies of diagnostic tests. Lijmer et al[3] and Rutjes et al[4] collected meta-analyses of diagnostic tests and examined what aspects of study design influenced the apparent diagnostic power of the tests. Whiting et al[5] systematically collected and reviewed *primary studies* that investigated the effects of bias on estimates of diagnostic test performances.

All 3 studies documented substantial bias associated with unrepresentative patient selection. Enrolling target-positive (those with the underlying condition of interest—in our scenario, people with dementia) and target-negative patients (those without the target condition) from separate populations results in overestimates of the test's power (*relative diagnostic odds ratio* [*RDOR*], 3.0; 95% confidence interval [CI], 2.0-4.5; and RDOR, 4.9; 95% CI, 0.6-37.3).[3,4] Even if investigators enroll target-positive and target-negative patients from the same population, nonconsecutive patient sampling and retrospective data collection may inflate estimates of diagnostic test performances (RDOR, 1.5; 95% CI, 1.0-2.1; and RDOR, 1.6; 95% CI, 1.1-2.2, respectively).[2,3] We label studies with unrepresentative patient selection as having spectrum bias. Table 12-2 summarizes the empirically supported sources of bias in studies of diagnostic tests.

Did the Investigators Compare the Test to an Appropriate, Independent Reference Standard?

The accuracy of a diagnostic test is best determined by comparing it to the "truth." Readers must assure themselves that investigators have applied an appropriate *reference*, *criterion*, or *gold standard* (such as biopsy, surgery, autopsy, or long-term follow-up without treatment) to every patient who undergoes the test under investigation.

TABLE 12-2

Empirical Evidence of Sources of Bias in Diagnostic Accuracy Studies[a]

	Lijmer et al[3] (RDOR; 95% CI)	Whiting et al[5]	Rutjes et al[4] (RDOR; 95% CI)
Did participating patients present a diagnostic dilemma?	Case-control design (3.0; 2.0-4.5)	Distorted selection of participants (some empirical support)	Case-control design (4.9; 0.6-37.3)
	Nonconsecutive patient selection (0.9; 0.7-1.1)		Nonconsecutive sampling (1.5; 1.0-2.1)
	Retrospective data collection (1.0; 0.7-1.4)		Retrospective data collection (1.6; 1.1-2.2)
Did investigators compare the test to an appropriate, independent reference standard?		Inappropriate reference standard (some empirical support)	
		Incorporation bias (using test as part of reference standard) (no empirical support)	Incorporation (1.4; 0.7-2.8)
Were those interpreting the test and reference standard blind to the other result	Not blinded (1.3; 1.0-1.9)	Review bias (some empirical support)	Single or non-blinded reading (1.1; 0.8-1.6)

(Continued)

TABLE 12-2

Empirical Evidence of Sources of Bias in Diagnostic Accuracy Studies[a] (Continued)

	Lijmer et al[3] (RDOR; 95% CI)	Whiting et al[5]	Rutjes et al[4] (RDOR; 95% CI)
Did investigators perform the same reference standard to all patients regardless of the results of the test under investigation?	Different reference tests (2.2; 1.5-3.3)	Differential verification bias (some empirical support)	Differential verification (1.6; 0.9-2.9)
	Partial verification (1.0; 0.8-1.3)	Partial verification bias (strong empirical support)	Partial verification (1.1; 0.7-1.7)

Abbreviations: CI, confidence interval; RDOR, relative diagnostic odds ratio.

[a]RDOR, point estimates, and 95% CIs are shown.

One way a study can go wrong is if the test that is being evaluated is part of the reference standard. The incorporation of the test into the reference standard is likely to inflate the estimate of the test's diagnostic power. Thus, clinicians should insist on the independence as one criterion for a satisfactory reference standard.

For instance, consider a study that evaluated the utility of abdominojugular reflux for the diagnosis of congestive heart failure. This study used, however, clinical and radiographic criteria, including abdominojugular reflex, as the reference test.[6] Another example comes from a study evaluating screening instruments for depression in terminally ill people. The authors claimed perfect performance (sensitivity = 1.0, specificity = 1.0) for a single question (Are you depressed?) to detect depression. Their diagnostic criteria included 9 questions, of which 1 was "Are you depressed?"[7]

In reading articles about diagnostic tests, if you cannot accept the reference standard (within reason, that is; after all, nothing is perfect), then the article is unlikely to provide valid results (Table 12-2).[4]

Were Those Interpreting the Test and Reference Standard Blind to the Other Results?

If you accept the reference standard, the next question is whether the interpreters of the test and reference standard were aware of the results of the other investigation (blind assessment).

Consider how, once clinicians see a pulmonary nodule on a computed tomographic (CT) scan, they can see the previously undetected lesion on the chest radiograph, or, once they learn the results of an echocardiogram, they hear a previously inaudible cardiac murmur.

The more likely that knowledge of the reference standard result can influence the interpretation of a test, the greater the importance of the blinded interpretation. Similarly, the more susceptible the reference standard is to changes in interpretation as a result of knowledge of the test being evaluated, the more important the blinding of the reference standard interpreter. The empirical study by Lijmer et al[3] demonstrated bias associated with unblinding, although the magnitude was small (RDOR, 1.3; 95% CI, 1.0-1.9), whereas Rutjes et al[4] found a compatible although statistically nonsignificant RDOR (RDOR, 1.1; 95% CI, 0.8-1.6) (Table 12-2).

Did Investigators Perform the Same Reference Standard to All Patients Regardless of the Results of the Test Under Investigation?

The properties of a diagnostic test will be distorted if its results influence whether patients undergo confirmation by the reference standard (verification[8,9] or work-up[10,11] bias). This can occur in 2 ways. First, only a selected sample of patients who underwent the index test may be verified by the reference standard. For example, patients with suspected coronary artery disease whose exercise test results are positive may be more likely to undergo coronary angiography (the reference standard) than those whose exercise test results are negative. Whiting et al[5] reviewed several documented instances of this type of verification bias, known as partial verification bias.

Second, results of the index test may be verified by different reference standards. Lijmer et al[3] and Rutjes et al[4] found a large magnitude of bias associated with the use of different reference tests for positive and negative results. The RDOR for this type of bias, also known as differential verification bias, was 2.2; 95% CI, 1.5-3.3[3] and 1.6; 95% CI, 0.9-2.9[4], respectively, in these 2 *systematic* reviews (Table 12-2).

Verification bias proved a problem for the Prospective Investigation of Pulmonary Embolism Diagnosis (PIOPED) study that evaluated the utility of ventilation perfusion scanning in the diagnosis of pulmonary embolism. Patients whose ventilation perfusion scan results were interpreted as "normal/near normal" and "low probability" were less likely to undergo pulmonary angiography (69%) than those with more positive ventilation perfusion scan results (92%), which is not surprising because clinicians might be reluctant to subject patients with a low probability of pulmonary embolism to the risks of angiography.[12]

Most articles would stop here, and readers would have to conclude that the magnitude of the bias resulting from different proportions of patients with high- and low-probability ventilation perfusion scans undergoing adequate angiography is uncertain but perhaps large. The PIOPED investigators, however, applied a second reference standard to the 150 patients with low-probability or normal/near-normal scan results who failed to undergo angiography (136 patients) or for whom angiogram interpretation was uncertain (14 patients). They judged such patients to be free of pulmonary embolism if they did well without treatment. Accordingly, they followed all such patients for 1 year without treating them with anticoagulant drugs. No patient developed clinically evident pulmonary embolism during follow-up, allowing us to conclude that patient-important pulmonary embolism (if we define patient-important pulmonary embolism as requiring anticoagulation therapy to prevent subsequent adverse events) was not present when they underwent ventilation perfusion scanning. Thus, the PIOPED study achieved the goal of applying a reference standard assessment to all patients but failed to apply the same standard to all.

USING THE GUIDE

The study of a brief diagnostic test for cognitive impairment included 2 cohorts. One was a stratified random sample of community-dwelling black persons aged 65 years and older; the other was a consecutive sample of nonselected nonscreened patients referred by family, caregivers, or providers for cognitive evaluation at the Alzheimer Disease Center. In the former group, the authors included all patients with a high suspicion of dementia on a detailed screening test and a random sample of those with moderate and low suspicion. The investigators faced diagnostic uncertainty in both populations. The populations are not perfect: the former included individuals without any suspicion of dementia, and the latter had already passed an initial screen at the primary care level (indeed, whether to refer for full geriatric assessment is one of the questions you are trying to resolve for the patient who triggered your literature search). Fortunately, test properties proved similar in the 2 populations, considerably lessening your concern.

All patients received the SIS, which asks the patient to remember 3 words (apple, table, penny); then to say the day of the week, month, and year; and finally to recall the 3 words without prompts. The number of errors provides a result with a range of 0 to 6.

For the reference standard diagnosis of dementia, patients had to satisfy both *Diagnostic and Statistical Manual of Mental Disorders* (Third Edition Revised) (*DSM-III-R*) and *International Classification of Diseases*, Tenth Revision (*ICD-10*) criteria, according to an assessment by a geriatric psychiatrist or a neurologist that included medical history and physical and neurologic examination; a complete neuropsychological test battery, including MMSE and 5 other tests; and interview with a relative of the participant.

Although you are satisfied with this reference standard, the published article leaves you unsure whether those making the SIS and the reference diagnosis were blind to the other results. To resolve the question, you e-mail the first author and ask for clarification. A couple of e-mails later, you have learned that "research assistants who had been trained and tested" administered the neuropsychological battery. On the other hand, "a consensus team composed of a geriatric psychiatrist, social psychologist, a geriatrician, and a neuropsychologist" made the reference standard diagnoses. The author reports that "there were open discussions of the case, and they had access to the entire medical record, including results of neuropsychological testing, at their disposal." The 6 items included in the SIS are derived from the MMSE but "were not pulled out as a separate instrument in the consensus team conference."

Thus, although there was no blinding, you suspect that this did not create important bias and are therefore ready to consider its results.

WHAT ARE THE RESULTS?

What Likelihood Ratios Were Associated With the Range of Possible Test Results?

In deciding how to interpret diagnostic tests results, we will consider its ability to change our estimate of the likelihood the patient has the target condition (we call this the pretest probability) to a more accurate estimate (we call this the posttest probability of the target disorder). The *likelihood ratio* (*LR*) for a particular test result moves us from the pretest probability to a posttest probability.

Put yourself in the place of the primary care physician in the scenario and consider 2 patients with suspected cognitive impairment with clear consciousness. The first is the 70-year-old woman in the clinical scenario who seems to be managing rather well but has a specific complaint that her memory is not what it used to be. The other is an 85-year-old woman, another longstanding patient, who arrives accompanied, for the first time, by her son. The concerned son tells you that she has, on one of her usual morning walks, lost her way. A neighbor happened to catch her a few miles away from home and notified him of the incident. On visiting his mother's house, he was surprised to find her room in a mess. Yet in your office, she greets you politely and protests that she was just having a bad day and does not think the incident warrants any fuss (at which point the son looks to the ceiling in frustrated disbelief). Your clinical hunches about the probability of dementia for these 2 people—that is, their pretest probabilities—are different. For the first woman, the probability is relatively low, perhaps 20%; for the second, it is relatively high, perhaps 70%.

The results of a formal screening test, the SIS in our example, will not tell us definitively whether dementia is present; rather, the results modify the pretest probability of that condition, yielding a new posttest probability. The direction and magnitude of this change from pretest to posttest probability are determined by the test's properties, and the property of most value is the LR.

We will use the results of the study by Callahan et al[1] to illustrate LRs. Table 12-3 presents the distribution of SIS scores in cohort of patients in the study by Callahan et al.[1]

How likely is a test result of 6 among people who do have dementia? Table 12-3 shows that 105 of 345 (or 30.4%) people with the condition made 6 errors. We can also see that of 306 people without dementia, 2 (or 0.65%) made 6 errors. How likely is this test result (ie, making 6 errors) in someone with dementia as opposed to someone without? Determining this requires us to look at the ratio of the 2 likelihoods that we have just calculated (30.4/0.65) and equals 47. In other words, the test result of 6 is 47 times as likely to occur in a patient with, as opposed to without, dementia.

TABLE 12-3

Six-Item Screener Scores in Patients With and Without Dementia, and Corresponding Likelihood Ratios

	Dementia (+)	Dementia (−)	Likelihood Ratio
SIS = 6	105	2	47
SIS = 5	64	2	28
SIS = 4	64	8	7.1
SIS = 3	45	16	2.5
SIS = 2	31	35	0.79
SIS = 1	25	80	0.28
SIS = 0	11	163	0.06
Sum	345	306	

Abbreviation: SIS, Six-Item Screener.

Data from Callahan et al.[1]

In a similar fashion, we can calculate the LR associated with a test result of each score. For example, the LR for the test score of 5 is (64/345)/(2/306) = 28. Table 12-3 provides the LR for each possible SIS score.

How can we interpret LRs? LRs indicate the extent to which a given diagnostic test result will increase or decrease the pretest probability of the target disorder. An LR of 1 tells us that the posttest probability is exactly the same as the pretest probability. LRs greater than 1.0 increase the probability that the target disorder is present; the higher the LR, the greater this increase. Conversely, LRs less than 1.0 decrease the probability of the target disorder, and the smaller the LR, the greater the decrease in probability.

How big is a "big" LR, and how small is a "small" one? Using LRs in your day-to-day practice will lead to your own sense of their interpretation, but consider the following a rough guide:

- LRs of greater than 10 or less than 0.1 generate large and often conclusive changes from pretest to posttest probability;

- LRs of 5 to 10 and 0.1 to 0.2 generate moderate shifts in pretest to posttest probability;

- LRs of 2 to 5 and 0.5 to 0.2 generate small (but sometimes important) changes in probability; and

- LRs of 1 to 2 and 0.5 to 1 alter probability to a small (and rarely important) degree.

Having determined the magnitude and significance of LRs, how do we use them to go from pretest to posttest probability? One way is to convert pretest probability to odds, multiply the result by the LR, and convert the consequent posttest odds into a posttest probability. A much easier strategy uses a nomogram proposed by Fagan[13] (Figure 12-1) that does all the conversions and allows an easy transition from pretest to posttest probability.

The left-hand column of this nomogram represents the pretest probability, the middle column represents the LR, and the right-hand column shows the posttest probability. You obtain the posttest probability by anchoring a ruler at the pretest probability and rotating it until it lines up with the LR for the observed test result. There is also a Web-based interactive program (http://www.JAMAevidence.com) that will do this for you. You can enter exact numbers for a pretest probability and an LR to obtain the exact posttest probability.

Recall the elderly woman from the opening scenario who has suspected dementia. We have decided that the probability of this patient's having the condition is about 20%. Let us suppose that the patient made 5 errors on the SIS. Anchoring a ruler at her pretest probability of 20% and aligning it with the LR of 28 associated with the test result of 5, you can obtain her posttest probability, around 90%.

The pretest probability is an estimate. Although the literature dealing with differential diagnosis can sometimes help us in

FIGURE 12-1

Likelihood Ratio Nomogram

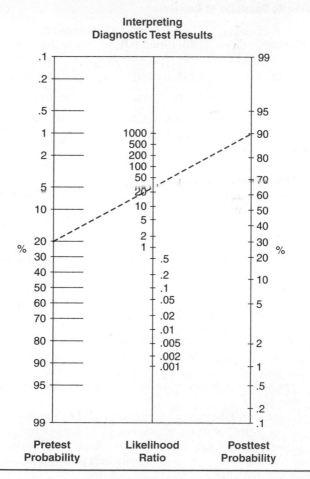

Interpreting
Diagnostic Test Results

Pretest
Probability

Likelihood
Ratio

Posttest
Probability

TABLE 12-4

Pretest Probabilities, Likelihood Ratios of the Six-Item Screener, and Posttest Probabilities in the 70-Year-Old Woman With Moderate Suspicion of Dementia

Pretest Probability, % (Range)[a]	SIS Result (LR)	Posttest Probability, % (Range)[a]
20 (10-30)	SIS = 6 (47)	92 (84-95)
	SIS = 5 (28)	88 (76-92)
	SIS = 4 (7.1)	64 (44-75)
	SIS = 3 (2.5)	38 (22-52)
	SIS = 2 (0.79)	16 (8-25)
	SIS = 1 (0.28)	7 (3-11)
	SIS = 0 (0.06)	1 (1-3)

Abbreviations: LR, likelihood ratio; SIS, Six-Item Screener.

[a]The values in parentheses represent a plausible range of *pretest probabilities*; that is, although the best guess as to the pretest probability is 20%, values of 10% to 30% would also be reasonable estimates.

establishing the pretest probability (see Chapter 11, Differential Diagnosis), we know of no such study that will complement our intuition in arriving at a pretest probability when the suspicion of dementia arises. Although our intuition makes precise estimates of pretest probability difficult, we can deal with residual uncertainty by examining the implications of a plausible range of pretest probabilities.

For example, if the pretest probability in this case is as low as 10% or as high as 30%, using the nomogram, we will obtain the posttest probability of about 80% and above 90%. Table 12-4 tabulates the posttest probabilities corresponding with each possible SIS score for the 70-year-old woman in the clinical scenario.

We can repeat this exercise for our second patient, the 85-year-old woman who had lost her way. You estimate that her history and presentation are compatible with a 70% probability of dementia. Using our nomogram (see Figure 12-1), the posttest probability with an SIS score of 6 or 5 is almost 100%; with an SIS score of 4, it is 94%; with an SIS score of 3, it is 85% and so on. The pretest probability (with a range of possible pretest probabilities from 60% to 80%), LRs, and posttest probabilities associated with each of these possible SIS scores are presented in Table 12-5.

Having learned to use LRs, you may be curious about where to find easy access to the LRs of the tests you use regularly in your own practice. The Rational Clinical Examination[14] is a series of *systematic reviews* of the diagnostic properties of the history and physical examination that have been published in *JAMA*. Further examples are accumulated on the *Users' Guides* Web site (http://www.JAMAevidence.com).

TABLE 12-5

Pretest Probabilities, Likelihood Ratios[a] of the Six-Item Screener, and Posttest Probabilities in the 85-Year-Old Woman With High Suspicion of Dementia

Pretest Probability, % (Range)[a]	SIS Result (LR)	Posttest Probability, % (Range)[a]
70 (60-80)	SIS = 6 (47)	99 (99-99)
	SIS = 5 (28)	98 (98-99)
	SIS = 4 (7.1)	94 (91-97)
	SIS = 3 (2.5)	85 (79-76)
	SIS = 2 (0.79)	65 (54-76)
	SIS = 1 (0.28)	40 (30-53)
	SIS = 0 (0.06)	12 (8-19)

Abbreviations: LR, Likelihood Ratio; SIS, Six-item Screener.

[a]The values in parentheses represent a plausible range of pretest probabilities. That is, although the best guess as to the pretest probability is 70%, values of 60% to 80% would also be reasonable estimates.

Dichotomizing Continuous Test Scores, Sensitivity and Specificity, and LR+ and LR–

Readers who have followed the discussion to this point will understand the essentials of interpretation of diagnostic tests. In part because they remain in wide use, it is also helpful to understand 2 other terms in the lexicon of diagnostic testing: *sensitivity* and *specificity*. Many articles on diagnostic tests report a 2 × 2 table and its associated sensitivity and specificity, as in Table 12-6, and to go along with it a figure that depicts the overall power of the diagnostic test (called a *receiver operating characteristic* [*ROC*] *curve*).

The study by Callahan et al[1] recommends a cutoff of 3 or more errors for the diagnosis of dementia. Table 12-7 provides the breakdown of the cohort of referred patients according to this cutoff.

TABLE 12-6

Comparison of the Results of a Diagnostic Test With the Results of Reference Standard Using a 2 × 2 Table

Test Results	Disease Present	Disease Absent
Test positive	TP	FP
Test negative	FN	TN

Sensitivity (Sens) $= \dfrac{TP}{TP + FN}$

Specificity (Spec) $= \dfrac{TN}{FP + TN}$

Likelihood ratio for positive test (LR+) $= \dfrac{Sens}{1 - Spec} = \dfrac{\text{True positive rate}}{\text{False positive rate}} = \dfrac{TP/(TP + FN)}{FP/(FP + TN)}$

Likelihood ratio for negative test (LR–) $= \dfrac{1 - Sens}{Spec} = \dfrac{\text{False negative rate}}{\text{True negative rate}} = \dfrac{FN/(TP + FN)}{TN/(FP + TN)}$

Abbreviation: FN, false negative; FP, false positive; TN, true negative; TP, true positive.

Sensitivity is the proportion of people with a positive test result among those with the target condition. Specificity is the proportion of people with a negative test result among those without the target condition.

TABLE 12-7

Comparison of the Results of a Diagnostic Test (Six-Item Screener) With the Results of Reference Standard (Consensus *DSM-IV* and *ICD-10* Diagnosis) Using the Recommended Cutoff

	Dementia (+)	Dementia (−)
SIS ≥ 3	278	28
SIS < 3	67	278
Sum	345	306

Abbreviation: *DSM-IV, Diagnostic and Statistical Manual of Mental Disorders*, (Fourth Edition); *ICD-10, International Classification of Diseases, Tenth Revision*; SIS, Six-Item Screener.

When we set the cutoff of 3 or more, SIS has a sensitivity of 0.81 (278/345) and a specificity of 0.91 (278/306). We can also calculate the LRs, exactly as we did in Table 12-3. The LR for SIS greater than or equal to 3 is therefore (278/345)/(28/306) = 8.8, and the LR for SIS less than 3 is (67/345)/(278/306) = 0.21. LR for a positive test result is often denoted as LR+, and that for a negative test result is denoted as LR−.

Let us now try to resolve our clinical scenario using this dichotomized 2 × 2 table. We had supposed that the pretest probability for the woman in the opening scenario was 20%, and she had made 5 errors. Because the SIS score of 5 is associated here with an LR+ of 8.8, using Fagan's nomogram,[13] we arrive at the posttest probability of around 70%, a figure considerably lower than the 90% that we had arrived at when we had a specific LR for 5 errors. This is because the dichotomized LR+ for SIS scores of 3 or more pooled strata for SIS scores of 3, 4, 5, and 6, and the resultant LR is thus diluted by the adjacent strata.

Although the difference between 70% and 90% may not dictate change in management strategies for the case in the clinical scenario, this will not always be the case. Consider a third patient, an elderly man with a pretest probability of 50% of dementia who has surprised us by making not a single error on the SIS. With the dichotomous LR+/LR− approach (or, for that matter, with the sensitivity/specificity approach, because these are mathematically equivalent and interchangeable), you combine the pretest probability of 50% with the LR– of 0.21 and arrive at the posttest probability of about 20%, likely necessitating further neuropsychological and other examinations. The true posttest probability for this man when we apply the LR associated with a score of 0 from Table 12-3 (0.06) is only about 5%. With this posttest probability, you (and the patient and his family) can feel relieved and be spared of further testing and further distress.

In summary, using multiple cuts or thresholds (sometimes referred to as multilevel LRs or stratum-specific LRs) has 2 key advantages over the sensitivity/specificity approach. First, for a test that produces continuous scores or a number of categories (which many tests in medicine do), using multiple thresholds retains as much information as possible. Second, knowing the LR of a particular test result, you can use a simple nomogram to move from the pretest to the posttest probability that is linked to your patient.

USING THE GUIDE

Thus far, we have established that the results are likely true for the people who were included in the study, and we have calculated the multilevel LRs associated with each possible score of the test. We have shown how the results could be applied to our patient (though we do not yet know the patient's score and have not decided how to proceed when we do).

HOW CAN I APPLY THE RESULTS TO PATIENT CARE?

Will the Reproducibility of the Test Result and Its Interpretation Be Satisfactory in My Clinical Setting?

The value of any test depends on its ability to yield the same result when reapplied to stable patients. Poor reproducibility can result from problems with the test itself (eg, variations in reagents in radioimmunoassay kits for determining hormone levels) or from its interpretation (eg, the extent of ST-segment elevation on an electrocardiogram). You can easily confirm this when you recall the clinical disagreements that arise when you and 1 or more colleagues examine the same electrocardiogram, ultrasonograph, or CT scan (even when all of you are experts).

Ideally, an article about a diagnostic test will address the reproducibility of the test results using a measure that corrects for agreement by chance, especially for issues of interpretation.

If the reported reproducibility of a test in the study setting is mediocre and disagreement between observers is common, and yet the test still discriminates well between those with and without the target condition, the test is likely to be useful. Under these circumstances, the likelihood is good that the test can be readily applied to your clinical setting.

If, on the other hand, reproducibility of a diagnostic test is high, either the test is simple and unambiguous or those interpreting it are highly skilled. If the latter applies, less skilled interpreters in your own clinical setting may not do as well. You will either need to obtain appropriate training (or ensure that those interpreting the test in your setting have that training) or look for an easier and more robust test.

Are the Study Results Applicable to the Patients in My Practice?

Test properties may change with a different mix of disease severity or with a different distribution of competing conditions. When patients with the target disorder all have severe disease, LRs will move away from a value of 1.0 (ie, sensitivity increases). If patients are all mildly affected, LRs move toward a value of 1.0 (ie, sensitivity decreases). If patients without the target disorder have competing conditions that mimic the test results observed for patients who do have the target disorder, the LRs will move closer to 1.0 and the test will appear less useful (ie, specificity decreases). In a different clinical setting in which fewer of the disease-free patients have these competing conditions, the LRs will move away from 1.0 and the test will appear more useful (ie, specificity increases).

Investigators have demonstrated the phenomenon of differing test properties in different subpopulations for exercise electrocardiography in the diagnosis of coronary artery disease. The more extensive the severity of coronary artery disease, the larger the LRs of abnormal exercise electrocardiography for angiographic narrowing of the coronary arteries.[15] Another example comes from the diagnosis of venous thromboembolism, in which compression ultrasonography for proximal-vein thrombosis has proved more accurate in symptomatic outpatients than in asymptomatic postoperative patients.[16]

Sometimes, a test fails in just the patients one hopes it will best serve. The LR of a negative dipstick test result for the rapid diagnosis of urinary tract infection is approximately 0.2 in patients with clear symptoms and thus a high probability of urinary tract infection but is more than 0.5 in those with low probability,[17] rendering it of little help in ruling out infection in the latter situation.

If you practice in a setting similar to that of the study, and if the patient under consideration meets all the study eligibility criteria, you can be confident that the results are applicable. If not, you must make a judgment. As with therapeutic interventions, you should ask whether there are compelling reasons why the results should not be applied to the patients in your practice, either because of the severity of disease in those patients or because the mix of competing conditions is so different that generalization is unwarranted. You may resolve the issue of generalizability if you can find an overview that summarizes the results of a number of studies.[18]

Will the Test Results Change My Management Strategy?

It is useful, when making and communicating management decisions, to link them explicitly to the probability of the target disorder. For any target disorder, there are probabilities below which a clinician would dismiss a diagnosis and order no further tests—the test threshold. Similarly, there are probabilities above which a clinician would consider the diagnosis confirmed and would stop testing and initiate treatment—the treatment threshold. When the probability of the target disorder lies between the test and treatment thresholds, further testing is mandated (see Chapter 10, The Process of Diagnosis).

If most patients have test results with LRs near 1.0, test results will seldom move us across the test or treatment threshold. Thus, the usefulness of a diagnostic test is strongly influenced by the proportion of patients suspected of having the target disorder whose test results have very high or very low LRs. Among the patients suspected of having dementia, a review of Table 12-3 allows us to determine the proportion of patients with extreme results (either LR > 10 or LR < 0.1). The proportion can be calculated as (105 + 2 + 64 + 2 + 11 + 163)/(345 + 306) or 347/651 = 53%. The SIS is likely to move the posttest probability in a decisive manner in half of the patients suspected of having dementia and examined, an impressive proportion and better than for most of our diagnostic tests.

A final comment has to do with the use of sequential tests. A new test can be integrated into the existing diagnostic pathway in 3 main ways—as replacement, triage, or add-on (Figure 12-2). That is, a new test can replace an existing test in the existing diagnostic pathway, can be performed before the old test so that only patients

FIGURE 12-2

Three Roles of a New Test in the Existing Diagnostic Pathway

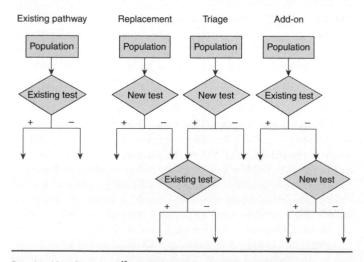

Reproduced from Bossuyt et al,[19] with permission from the BMJ Publishing Group.

with particular results on this triage test continue the testing pathway, or can be placed after the old test so that only patients with a particular result on the old test may need this add-on new test.[19]

The LR approach fits in particularly well in thinking about the diagnostic pathway. Each item of the medical history, or each finding on physical examination, represents a diagnostic test. We can use one test to obtain a certain posttest probability that can be further increased or decreased by using another subsequent test. In general, we can also use laboratory tests or imaging procedures in the same way. If 2 tests are closely related, however, application of the second test may provide little or no information, and the sequential application of LRs will yield misleading results. For example, once one has the results of the most powerful laboratory test for iron deficiency, serum ferritin, additional tests such as serum iron or transferrin saturation add no further useful information.[20]

Clinical prediction rules deal with the lack of independence of a series of tests and provide the clinician with a way of combining their results. For instance, for patients with suspected pulmonary embolism, one could use a rule that incorporates respiratory symptoms, heart rate, leg symptoms, oxygen saturation, electrocardiographic findings, and other aspects of medical history and physical examination to accurately classify patients with suspected pulmonary embolism as being characterized by high, medium, and low probability.[21]

Will Patients Be Better Off as a Result of the Test?

The ultimate criterion for the usefulness of a diagnostic test is whether the benefits that accrue to patients are greater than the associated risks.[22] How can we establish the benefits and risks of applying a diagnostic test? The answer lies in thinking of a diagnostic test as a therapeutic maneuver (see Chapter 6, Therapy). Establishing whether a test does more good than harm will involve randomizing patients to a diagnostic strategy that includes the test under investigation, creating a management schedule linked to the diagnostic strategy or to one in which the test is not available, and following up patients in both groups to determine the frequency of patient-important outcomes.

When is demonstrating accuracy sufficient to mandate the use of a test, and when does one require a randomized controlled trial? The value of an accurate test will be undisputed when the target disorder is dangerous if left undiagnosed, if the test has acceptable risks, and if effective treatment exists. This is the case for the ventilation perfusion scan for suspected pulmonary embolism. A high-probability or normal/near-normal result of a ventilation perfusion scan may well eliminate the need for further investigation and may result in anticoagulant agents being appropriately given or appropriately withheld (with either course of action having a substantial positive influence on patient outcome).

Sometimes, a test may be completely benign, represent a low resource investment, be evidently accurate, and clearly lead to useful changes in management. Such is the case for use of the SIS in patients with suspected dementia, when test results may dictate reassurance or extensive investigation and ultimately planning for a deteriorating course.

In other clinical situations, tests may be accurate, and management may even change as a result of their application, but their effect on patient outcome may be far less certain. Consider one of the issues we raised in our discussion of framing clinical questions (see Chapter 3, What Is the Question). There, we considered a patient with apparently resectable non–small-cell carcinoma of the lung and wondered whether the clinician should order a CT scan and base further management on the results or whether an immediate mediastinoscopy should be undertaken. For this question, knowledge of the accuracy of CT scanning is insufficient. A randomized trial of CT-directed management or mediastinoscopy for all patients is warranted, and indeed, investigators have conducted such a trial.[23] Other examples include catheterization of the right side of the heart for critically ill patients with uncertain hemodynamic status and bronchoalveolar lavage for critically ill patients with possible pulmonary infection. For these tests, randomized trials have helped elucidate optimal management strategies.

USING THE GUIDE

Although the study itself does not report reproducibility, its scoring is simple and straightforward because you need only count the number of errors made to 6 questions. It does not require any props or visual cues and is therefore unobtrusive and easy to administer. The SIS takes only 1 to 2 minutes to complete (compared with 5 to 10 minutes for the MMSE). The appendix of the published article gives a detailed word-by-word instruction on how to administer the SIS. You believe that you too can administer this scale reliably.

The patient in the clinical scenario is an older woman who was able to come to your clinic by herself but appeared no longer as lucid as she used to be. The Alzheimer Disease Center cohort in the study we had been examining in this chapter consists of people suspected of having dementia by their caregivers and brought to a tertiary care center directly. Their test characteristics were reported to be similar to those observed in the general population cohort, that is, in a sample with less severe presentations. You decide that there is no compelling reason that the study results would not apply to your patient.

You invite your patient back to the office for a follow-up visit and administer the SIS. The result is a score of 4, which, given your pretest probability of 20%, increases the probability to more than 60%. After hearing that you are concerned about her memory and possibly about her function, she agrees to a referral to a geriatrician for more extensive investigation.

References

1. Callahan CM, Unverzagt FW, Hui SL, Perkins AJ, Hendrie HC. Six-Item Screener to identify cognitive impairment among potential subjects for clinical research. *Med Care*. 2002;40(9):771-781.

2. Thomson DM, Krupey J, Freedman SO, Gold P. The radioimmunoassay of circulating carcinoembryonic antigen of the human digestive system. *Proc Natl Acad Sci U S A*. 1969;64(1):161-167.

3. Lijmer JG, Mol BW, Heisterkamp S, et al. Empirical evidence of design-related bias in studies of diagnostic tests. *JAMA*. 1999;282(11):1061-1066.

4. Rutjes AW, Reitsma JB, Di Nisio M, Smidt N, van Rijn JC, Bossuyt PM. Evidence of bias and variation in diagnostic accuracy studies. *CMAJ*. 2006;174(4):469-476.

5. Whiting P, Rutjes AW, Reitsma JB, Glas AS, Bossuyt PM, Kleijnen J. Sources of variation and bias in studies of diagnostic accuracy: a systematic review. *Ann Intern Med*. 2004;140(3):189-202.

6. Marantz PR, Kaplan MC, Alderman MH. Clinical diagnosis of congestive heart failure in patients with acute dyspnea. *Chest*. 1990;97(4):776-781.

7. Chochinov HM, Wilson KG, Enns M, Lander S. Are you depressed? screening for depression in the terminally ill. *Am J Psychiatry*. 1997;154(5):674-676.

8. Begg CB, Greenes RA. Assessment of diagnostic tests when disease verification is subject to selection bias. *Biometrics*. 1983;39(1):207-215.

9. Gray R, Begg CB, Greenes RA. Construction of receiver operating characteristic curves when disease verification is subject to selection bias. *Med Decis Making*. 1984;4(2):151-164.

10. Ransohoff DF, Feinstein AR. Problems of spectrum and bias in evaluating the efficacy of diagnostic tests. *N Engl J Med*. 1978;299(17):926-930.

11. Choi BC. Sensitivity and specificity of a single diagnostic test in the presence of work-up bias. *J Clin Epidemiol*. 1992;45(6):581-586.

12. PIOPED Investigators. Value of the ventilation/perfusion scan in acute pulmonary embolism: results of the Prospective Investigation of Pulmonary Embolism Diagnosis (PIOPED). *JAMA*. 1990;263(20):2753-2759.

13. Fagan TJ. Letter: nomogram for Bayes theorem. *N Engl J Med*. 1975;293 (5):257.

14. Sackett DL, Rennie D. The science of the art of the clinical examination. *JAMA*. 1992;267(19):2650-2652.

15. Hlatky MA, Pryor DB, Harrell FE Jr, Califf RM, Mark DB, Rosati RA. Factors affecting sensitivity and specificity of exercise electrocardiography: multivariable analysis. *Am J Med*. 1984;77(1):64-71.

16. Ginsberg JS, Caco CC, Brill-Edwards PA, et al. Venous thrombosis in patients who have undergone major hip or knee surgery: detection with compression US and impedance plethysmography. *Radiology*. 1991;181(3):651-654.

17. Lachs MS, Nachamkin I, Edelstein PH, Goldman J, Feinstein AR, Schwartz JS. Spectrum bias in the evaluation of diagnostic tests: lessons from the rapid dipstick test for urinary tract infection. *Ann Intern Med*. 1992;117(2):135-140.

18. Irwig L, Tosteson AN, Gatsonis C, et al. Guidelines for meta-analyses evaluating diagnostic tests. *Ann Intern Med*. 1994;120(8):667-676.

19. Bossuyt PM, Irwig L, Craig J, Glasziou P. Comparative accuracy: assessing new tests against existing diagnostic pathways. *BMJ*. 2006;332(7549):1089-1092.

20. Guyatt GH, Oxman AD, Ali M, Willan A, McIlroy W, Patterson C. Laboratory diagnosis of iron-deficiency anemia: an overview. *J Gen Intern Med*. 1992;7(2):145-153.

21. Wells PS, Ginsberg JS, Anderson DR, et al. Use of a clinical model for safe management of patients with suspected pulmonary embolism. *Ann Intern Med*. 1998;129(12):997-1005.

22. Guyatt GH, Tugwell PX, Feeny DH, Haynes RB, Drummond M. A framework for clinical evaluation of diagnostic technologies. *CMAJ*. 1986; 134(6):587-594.

23. Canadian Lung Oncology Group. Investigation for mediastinal disease in patients with apparently operable lung cancer. *Ann Thorac Surg*. 1995; 60(5):1382-1389.

PROGNOSIS

Adrienne Randolph, Deborah J. Cook,
and Gordon Guyatt

IN THIS CHAPTER:

Can I Use the Results in the Management of Patients in My Practice?

Clinical Resolution

CLINICAL SCENARIO

What Is the Prognosis of a Patient Aged 364 Days With Newly Diagnosed Neuroblastoma?

Three months into pediatric internship, you saw a clinic patient for her 12-month routine health checkup. Although she was healthy except for her big stomach, you felt something in the abdomen that you thought could be a tumor. During the next several weeks, the infant undergoes abdominal ultrasonography and magnetic resonance imaging, bone scintigraphy, a skeletal survey, and finally a bone marrow and tumor biopsy. The day after tomorrow is your patient's first birthday. You sat with the oncologist as she told the patient's family that their infant daughter has neuroblastoma, the most common intra-abdominal malignancy of infancy. The parents learn that, because the infant was younger than 365 days on the initial diagnosis and because her tumor markers and bone marrow involvement were consistent with stage IV-S disease and a favorable *prognosis*, she has at least an 85% chance of cure with surgical resection. The oncologist also told the parents that children older than 1 year with different tumor markers and extent of disease usually need additional chemotherapy and sometimes a bone marrow transplant. Still numb and trying to take it all in, the parents have no questions for the oncologist. Later, when you are following up with them in the family waiting area, they express worry that their infant daughter was diagnosed so close to the 365-day age cutoff. They ask you what would have happened if her checkup had been 3 weeks later, when it was originally scheduled. Would her prognosis then be worse? You see their point. Their doubt makes you wonder where the oncologist got the estimate of an 85% or higher cure. You decide to check out the *evidence* for yourself.

FINDING THE EVIDENCE

You use your hospital's free Internet connection to access MEDLINE at the National Library of Medicine Web site via PubMed. You click on the "Clinical Queries" section under PubMed services. Under the "Search by Clinical Study Category" section, you enter the terms "neuroblastoma" and "age" and click on "prognosis" and "narrow, specific search." You see an article titled "Evidence for an Age Cutoff Greater Than 365 Days for Neuroblastoma Risk Group Stratification in the Children's Oncology Group [COG]."[1] The librarian helps you to obtain a copy from the hospital library. This data analysis from multiple pediatric neuroblastoma clinical trials and *observational studies*, including 3666 children with neuroblastoma, examined the effect of age on the likelihood of recurrence.[1]

WHY AND HOW WE MEASURE PROGNOSIS

Clinicians help patients in 3 broad ways: by diagnosing what is wrong with them, by administering treatment that does more good than *harm*, and by giving them an indication of what the future is likely to hold. Clinicians require studies of *prognosis*—those examining the possible *outcomes* of a disease and the probability with which they can be expected to occur—to achieve the second and third goals.

Knowledge of a patient's prognosis can help clinicians make the right treatment decisions. If a patient will get well anyway, clinicians should not recommend expensive or potentially toxic treatments. If a patient is at low risk of adverse outcomes, even beneficial treatments may not be worthwhile. On the other hand, patients may be destined to have poor outcomes despite whatever treatment we offer. Aggressive therapy in such individuals may only prolong suffering and waste resources. Whatever the treatment possibilities, by understanding prognosis and presenting the expected future course of a patient's illness, clinicians also offer reassurance and hope, or preparation for death or long-term disability.

To estimate a patient's prognosis, we examine outcomes in groups of patients with a similar clinical presentation. We may then refine our prognosis by looking at subgroups defined by demographic variables such as age and by *comorbidity* and decide which subgroup the patient belongs in. When these variables or factors really do predict which patients do better or worse, we call them *prognostic factors*.

Authors may distinguish between prognostic factors and *risk factors*, those patient characteristics associated with the development of the disease in the first place. For example, smoking is an important risk factor for the development of lung cancer, but it is not an important prognostic factor in someone who has lung cancer. The issues in studies of prognostic factors and risk factors are identical for assessing *validity* and for using the results in patient care.

In this chapter, we focus on how to use articles that may contain valid prognostic information that physicians will find useful for counseling patients (Table 13-1).

TABLE 13-1

Users' Guides to an Article About Prognosis

Are the results valid?

- Was the sample of patients representative?
- Were the patients sufficiently homogeneous with respect to prognostic risk?
- Was follow-up sufficiently complete?
- Were outcome criteria objective and unbiased?

What are the results?

- How likely are the outcomes over time?
- How precise are the estimates of likelihood?

How can I apply the results to patient care?

- Were the study patients and their management similar to those in my practice?
- Was the follow-up sufficiently long?
- Can I use the results in the management of patients in my practice?

Using the same observational study (*cohort* and *case-control*) designs as investigators addressing issues of harm (see Chapter 9, Harm), investigators addressing issues of prognosis conduct studies to explore the determinants of outcome. Implicitly, *randomized controlled trials* also address issues of prognosis. The results reported for the treatment group and the *control group* both provide prognostic information: The control group results tell us about the prognosis in patients who did not receive the *experimental therapy*, whereas the experimental group results tell us about the prognosis in patients receiving the investigational intervention. In this sense, each arm of a randomized trial represents a cohort study. If the randomized trial meets the criteria we describe later in this chapter, it can provide useful information about patients' likely fate.

ARE THE RESULTS VALID?

Was the Sample of Patients Representative?

Bias has to do with systematic differences from the truth. A prognostic study is biased if it yields a systematic overestimate or underestimate of the likelihood of adverse outcomes in the patients under study. When a sample is systematically different from the population of interest and is therefore likely biased because patients will have a better or worse prognosis than those in the population of interest, we label the sample as unrepresentative.

How can you recognize an unrepresentative sample? First, determine whether patients pass through some sort of filter before entering the study. If they do, the result is likely a sample that is systematically different from the underlying population of interest. One such filter is the sequence of referrals that leads patients from primary to tertiary centers. Tertiary centers often care for patients with rare and unusual disorders or increased illness severity. Research describing the outcomes of patients in tertiary centers may not be applicable to the general patient with the disorder in the community (sometimes referred to as *referral bias*).

As an example, when children are admitted to the hospital with febrile seizures, parents want to know the risk of their child having more seizures. This risk is much lower in population-based studies (reported risks range from 1.5% to 4.6%) than in clinic-based studies (reported risks are 2.6% to 76.9%).[2] Those in clinic-based studies may have other neurologic problems predisposing them to have higher rates of recurrence.

Were the Patients Sufficiently Homogeneous With Respect to Prognostic Risk?

Prognostic studies are most useful if individual members of the entire group of patients being considered are similar enough that the outcome of the group is applicable to each group member. This will be true only if patients are at a similar well-described point in their disease process. The point in the clinical course need not be early, but it does need to be consistent. For instance, in a study of the prognosis of children with acquired brain injury, researchers examined not the entire population but a subpopulation that remained unconscious after 90 days.[3]

After ensuring that patients were at the same disease stage, you must consider other factors that might influence patient outcome. If factors such as age or severity influence prognosis, then providing a single prognosis for young and old, mild and severe, will be misleading for each of these subgroups. For instance, a study examining neurologic outcome in children with acquired brain injury that pooled patients with and without head trauma would mislead if these 2 groups have different prognoses. Indeed, the authors of a study addressing the issue[3] found that patients with posttraumatic injuries fared much better than those with anoxic injuries. Of 36 patients with closed head injury, 23 (64%) regained enough social function to express their wants and needs and 9 (25%) eventually regained the capacity to walk independently. Of 13 children with anoxic injuries, none regained important social or cognitive function. Providing an overall intermediate prognosis for both groups would profoundly mislead the parents of these children.

Not only must investigators consider all important prognostic factors but also they must consider them in relation to one another.

If sickness but not age truly determines outcome, and sicker patients tend to be older, investigators who fail to simultaneously consider age and severity of illness may mistakenly conclude that age is an important prognostic factor. For example, investigators in the Framingham study examined risk factors for stroke.[4] They reported that the rate of stroke in patients with atrial fibrillation and rheumatic heart disease was 41 per 1000 person-years, which was similar to the rate for patients with atrial fibrillation but without rheumatic heart disease. Patients with rheumatic heart disease were, however, much younger than those who did not have rheumatic heart disease. To properly understand the influence of rheumatic heart disease, investigators in these circumstances must consider separately the relative risk of stroke in young people with and without rheumatic disease and the risk of stroke in elderly people with and without rheumatic disease. We call this separate consideration an *adjusted analysis*. Once adjustments were made for age, the investigators found that the rate of stroke was 6-fold greater in patients with rheumatic heart disease and atrial fibrillation than in patients with atrial fibrillation who did not have rheumatic heart disease.

If a large number of variables have a major effect on prognosis, investigators should use sophisticated statistical techniques such as regression analysis to determine the most powerful predictors. Such an analysis may lead to a *clinical decision rule* that guides clinicians in simultaneously considering all of the important prognostic factors.

How can you decide whether the groups are sufficiently homogeneous with respect to their risk? On the basis of your clinical experience and your understanding of the biology of the condition under study, can you think of factors that the investigators have neglected that are likely to define subgroups with very different prognoses? To the extent that the answer is yes, the validity of the study results may be compromised.

Was Follow-up Sufficiently Complete?

Investigators who lose track of a large number of patients compromise the validity of their prognostic study. The reason is that those who are followed may be at systematically higher or lower risk than those not followed. As the number of patients who do not return for *follow-up* increases, the likelihood of bias also increases.

How many patients lost to follow-up is too many? The answer depends on the relationship between the proportion of patients who are lost and the proportion of patients who have had the adverse outcome of interest. The larger the number of patients whose fate is unknown relative to the number who have had the adverse event, the greater the threat to the study's validity. For instance, let us assume that 30% of a particularly high-risk group (such as elderly patients with diabetes) have had an adverse outcome (such as cardiovascular death) during long-term follow-up. If 10% of the patients have been lost to follow-up, the true rate of patients who had died may be as low as approximately 27% or as high as 37%. Across this range, the clinical implications would not change appreciably, and the loss to follow-up does not threaten the validity of the study. However, in a much lower-risk patient sample (otherwise healthy middle-aged patients, for instance), the observed event rate may be 1%. In this case, if we assumed that all 10% of the patients lost to follow-up had died, the event rate of 11% might have very different implications.

A large loss to follow-up constitutes a more serious threat to validity when the patients who are lost may be different from those who are easier to find. In one study, for example, after much effort, the investigators managed to follow 180 of 186 patients treated for neurosis.[5] The death rate was 3% among the 60% who were easily traced. Among those who were more difficult to find, however, the death rate was 27%.

If a differential fate for those followed and those lost is plausible (and in most prognostic studies, it will be), loss to follow-up that is large in relation to the proportion of patients having an adverse outcome of interest constitutes an important threat to validity.

Were Outcome Criteria Objective and Unbiased?

Outcome events may be objective and easily measured (eg, death), require some judgment (eg, myocardial infarction), or require considerable judgment and effort to measure (eg, disability, quality of life). Investigators should clearly specify and define their *target outcomes* and, whenever possible, they should base their criteria on objective measures.

The study of children with acquired brain injury provides a good example of the issues involved in measuring outcome.[3] The examiners found that patients' families frequently optimistically interpreted interactions with the patients. The investigators therefore required that development of a social response in the affected children be verified by study personnel.

USING THE GUIDE

Returning to our opening clinical scenario, the investigators in the COG neuroblastoma prognosis study used data from 3666 children younger than 21 years with a pathologically confirmed diagnosis of neuroblastoma who participated in 1 of 11 therapeutic trials or observational studies.[1] Because more than 60% of all children treated for cancer participate in clinical trials vs less than 2% of adult patients with cancer,[6] this cohort is likely to represent most of the children with neuroblastoma. The investigators considered whether subgroups defined by age, disease stage, and cancer stage and tumor marker (*MYCN*) amplification (a tumor marker that is either amplified or nonamplified) differed in their prognosis. The investigators do not report the number of patients lost to follow-up, and this is problematic. A review of the 5 references that included data from the 13 study reports reveals that some patients were registered for multiple studies with different follow-up requirements. It is not possible to determine the rate of loss to follow-up in the 3666 children from review of the referenced reports. Finally, the authors defined *event-free survival* as patients who were free of relapse of the cancer, disease progression, secondary malignancy, and death. Although death is an objective, straightforward outcome, identification of disease progression, secondary malignancy, and cancer relapse may have differed across the numerous studies. Although you have some reservations about completeness of long-term follow-up, you conclude that the study is still likely to provide a good estimate of the prognosis of the child under your care and should help you to address the parents' question.

WHAT ARE THE RESULTS?

How Likely Are the Outcomes Over Time?

Results from studies of prognosis or risk are the number of events that occur over time. An informative way to depict these results is a *survival curve*, which is a graph of the number of events over time (or conversely, the chance of being free of these events over time) (see Chapter 7, Does Treatment Lower Risk? Understanding the Results). The events must be yes/no (eg, death, stroke, recurrence of cancer), and investigators must know the time at which they occur. Figure 13-1 shows 2 survival curves, one of survival after a myocardial infarction[7]; the other, need for revision surgery after hip replacement surgery.[8]

The chance of dying after a myocardial infarction is highest shortly after the event (reflected by an initially steep downward slope of the curve, which then becomes flat), whereas few hip replacements require revision until much later (this curve, by contrast, starts out flat and then steepens).

FIGURE 13-1

Survival Curves

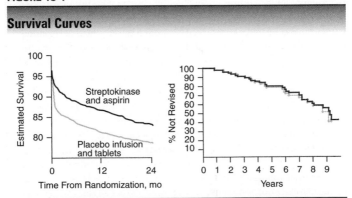

Left, Survival after myocardial infarction. Right, Results of hip replacement surgery: percentage of patients who survived without needing a new procedure (revision) after their initial hip replacement.

Reprinted from *The Lancet*,[7] Copyright © 1988, with permission from Elsevier (left). Reprinted from Dorey and Amstutz,[8] with permission from the *Journal of Bone and Joint Surgery* (right).

How Precise Are the Estimates of Likelihood?

The more precise the estimate of prognosis a study provides, the less we need be uncertain about the estimated prognosis and the more useful it is to us. Usually, authors report the risks of adverse outcomes with their associated 95% *confidence intervals* (*CIs*). If the study is valid, the 95% CI defines the range of risks within which it is highly likely that the true risk lies (see Chapter 8, Confidence Intervals). For example, a study of the prognosis of patients with dementia provided a 95% CI around the 49% estimate of survival at 5 years after presentation (ie, 39%-58%).[9]

In most survival curves, the earlier follow-up periods usually include results from more patients than do the later periods (owing to losses to follow-up and because patients are not enrolled in the study at the same time), which means that the survival curves are more precise in the earlier periods, indicated by narrower confidence bands around the lefthand parts of the curve (Figure 13-2).

USING THE GUIDE

The COG neuroblastoma study[1] evaluated the relative risk for an event in younger and older children before and after adjusting for *MYCN* status. You are concerned that, because your patient was diagnosed at about 365 days of age, she might be in a higher-risk group. Figure 13-3 shows the relevant results. Figure 13-3A shows that, before adjustment for stage and *MYCN* status, older age appears to have a large negative effect on prognosis. This is misleading, however, because older children also tend to have worse stage and marker status. Figure 13-3B shows a much more modest influence of age after adjustment. Note that the CIs are narrower in the younger age groups because most patients are diagnosed before 20 months of age. Figure 13-3B shows that risk begins to increase appreciably after 600, not 365, days.

FIGURE 13-2

Risk for an Event by Age Group in Children With Neuroblastoma

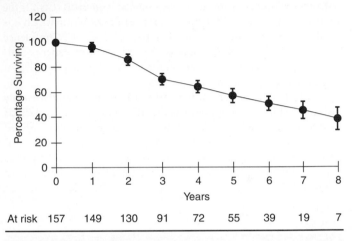

| At risk | 157 | 149 | 130 | 91 | 72 | 55 | 39 | 19 | 7 |

Reproduced from Wood et al,[10] with permission of Wiley-Liss, Inc, a subsidary of John Wiley & Sons, Inc. Copyright © 1999, American Cancer Society.

HOW CAN I APPLY THE RESULTS TO PATIENT CARE?

Were the Study Patients and Their Management Similar to Those in My Practice?

Authors should describe the study patients explicitly and in enough detail that you can make a comparison with your patients. One factor sometimes neglected in prognostic studies that could strongly influence outcome is therapy. Therapeutic strategies often vary markedly among institutions and change over time as new treatments become available or old treatments regain popularity. To the extent that treatments are beneficial or detrimental, overall patient outcome might improve or become worse.

FIGURE 13-3

Relative Risk for an Event, With 95% Confidence Intervals, by Age Group in Children With Neuroblastoma

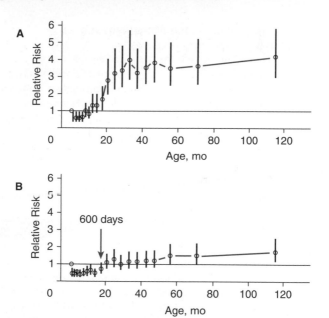

A, Univariate Cox proportional hazards model with age group. B, Multivariate Cox proportional model with International Neuroblastoma Staging System stage, MYCN status, and age group. There is neither increased nor decreased risk for an event where the curve crosses relative risk = 1 at roughly 600 days (19.7 months) of age. Reprinted from London et al,[1] with permission of the American Society of Clinical Oncology.

Reprinted from London et al,[1] with permission of the American Society of Clinical Oncology.

Was Follow-up Sufficiently Long?

Because the presence of illness often precedes the development of an outcome event by a long period, investigators must follow patients for a period long enough to detect the outcomes of interest. For example, recurrence in some women with early breast cancer can occur many years after initial diagnosis and treatment.[11] A prognostic study may

provide an unbiased assessment of outcome during a short period if it
meets the validity criteria in Table 13-1, but it may be of little use if a
patient is interested in her prognosis during a long period.

Can I Use the Results in the Management of Patients in My Practice?

Prognostic data often provide the basis for sensible decisions about
therapy. Even if the prognostic result does not help with selection of
appropriate therapy, it can help you in counseling a concerned
patient or relative. Some conditions, such as asymptomatic hiatal
hernia or asymptomatic colonic diverticulae, have such a good
overall prognosis that they have been termed *nondisease*.[12] On the
other hand, a result of uniformly bad prognosis could provide a
clinician with a starting place for a discussion with the patient and
family, leading to counseling about end-of-life care.

CLINICAL RESOLUTION

Your patient resembles those in the favorable risk subgroup of
children in the study[1] in age, stage, and tumor markers, and you
can readily generalize the results to her care. Therapeutic
management for patients with this risk profile across the studies
is similar to what your patient will receive. The minimal follow-
up in the study was 3 years, and half of the patients were
followed up to 5.8 years, allowing investigators to provide
estimates for patients up to 5 years after diagnosis, which you
consider adequate for advising the parents.

Although the parents are still upset abut the diagnosis of
neuroblastoma in their infant and have to come to grips with
any associated mortality risk, you have gleaned some reas-
suring information from the study.[1] All of your patient's
findings suggest the most favorable prognosis. The study tells
us that the 4-year event-free survival of patients 365 to 460
days old, excluding those with stage 4 disease and *MYCN*-amplified

tumors, is 92% ± 3% standard error. Table 13-2 shows how to calculate CIs from standard errors of a proportion, which for the study under consideration, with 135 patients in that subgroup, gives a CI of 91.6% to 92.4%. Given the narrow CIs, you are secure using these estimates. Although your patient is at the 365-day mark at presentation, it is clear that risk does not increase appreciably with age until after 600 days. Your patient is still in the most favorable risk group, and you can reassure the parents that toxic chemotherapy is not necessary at this point.

TABLE 13-2

Calculating 95% Confidence Intervals From a Proportion

I. The rule of 3s[13]

Used when the numerator is 0 or 1 and there are at least 30 patients in the sample

$= 100 \times 3$/number of patients = upper limit of the 95% CI

Example: 50 of 50 patients die; the upper limit of the 95% CI for survival $= 100 \times 3/50 = 6\%$, or given a sample size of 50, the survival rate could still be as high as 6%.

II. Calculating the 95% CI from the standard error of a proportion[14]

Used when 2 or more patients have the outcome of interest

p = proportion = number of patients with the outcome/total number of patients

sep = standard error of the proportion = square root of $[p \times (1 - p)]/n$.

95% CI $= 100 \times [p - (1.96 \times sep)], 100 \times [p + (1.96 \times sep)]$

Example from our scenario: 124 of 135 survive, $p = 0.92$, sep = square root of $(0.92 \times 0.08)/135 = 0.002$, $1.96 \times sep = 1.96 \times 0.002 = 0.004$, 95% CI $= 100 \times (0.92 - 0.004), 100 \times (0.92 + 0.004) = 91.6\%$ to 92.4%, which is the 95% CI.

Abbreviation: CI, confidence interval.

References

1. London WB, Castleberry RP, Matthay KK, et al. Evidence for an age cutoff greater than 365 days for neuroblastoma risk group stratification in the Children's Oncology Group. *J Clin Oncol.* 2005;23(27):6459-6465.

2. Ellenberg JH, Nelson KB. Sample selection and the natural history of disease: studies of febrile seizures. *JAMA.* 1980;243(13):1337-1340.

3. Kriel RL, Krach LE, Jones-Saete C. Outcome of children with prolonged unconsciousness and vegetative states. *Pediatr Neurol.* 1993;9(5):362-368.

4. Wolf PA, Dawber TR, Thomas HE Jr, et al. Epidemiologic assessment of chronic atrial fibrillation and risk of stroke: the Framingham study. *Neurology.* 1978;28(10):973-977.

5. Sims AC. Importance of a high tracing-rate in long-term medical follow-up studies. *Lancet.* 1973;2(7826):433-435.

6. Murthy VH, Krumholz HM, Gross CP. Participation in cancer clinical trials: race-, sex-, and age-based disparities. *JAMA.* 2004;291(22):2720-2726.

7. ISIS-2 (Second International Study of Infarct Survival) Collaborative Group. Randomised trial of intravenous streptokinase, oral aspirin, both, or neither among 17,187 cases of suspected acute myocardial infarction: ISIS-2. *Lancet.* 1988;2(8607):349-360.

8. Dorey F, Amstutz HC. The validity of survivorship analysis in total joint arthroplasty. *J Bone Joint Surg Am.* 1989;71(4):544-548.

9. Walsh JS, Welch HG, Larson EB. Survival of outpatients with Alzheimer-type dementia. *Ann Intern Med.* 1990;113(6):429-434.

10. Wood LA, Coupland RW, North SA, Palmer MC. Outcome of advanced stage low grade follicular lymphomas in a population-based retrospective cohort. *Cancer.* 1999;85(6):1361-1368.

11. Early Breast Cancer Trialists' Collaborative Group. Systemic treatment of early breast cancer by hormonal, cytotoxic, or immune therapy: 133 randomised trials involving 31,000 recurrences and 24,000 deaths among 75,000 women. *Lancet.* 1992;339(8784):1-15.

12. Meador CK. The art and science of nondisease. *N Engl J Med.* 1965 Jan 14; 272:92-95.

13. Hanley JA, Lippman-Hand A. If nothing goes wrong, is everything all right? interpreting zero numerators. *JAMA.* 1983;249(13):1743-1745.

14. Sackett DL, Haynes RB, Guyatt GH, Tugwell P, eds. Making a prognosis. In: *Clinical Epidemiology: A Basic Science for Clinical Medicine.* 2nd ed. Toronto, Ontario, Canada: Little, Brown & Company; 1991.

SUMMARIZING THE EVIDENCE

Gordon Guyatt, Roman Jaeschke,
Kameshwar Prasad, and Deborah J. Cook

IN THIS CHAPTER:

What Is the Overall Quality of the Evidence?

Are the Benefits Worth the Costs and Potential Risks?

Clinical Resolution

CLINICAL SCENARIO

Should We Administer Intravenous Magnesium to Patients Presenting With Acute Severe Asthma?

❶n call for general internal medicine, you receive a referral of a 26-year-old woman with asthma exacerbation. She was in the emergency department 2 weeks earlier and was discharged after treatment with brochodilators and prescription for a short course of oral steroids. Despite advice to do so, she has not been able to give up her new cat. Her forced expired volume in 1 second (FEV_1), 78% predicted when she departed the emergency department 2 weeks ago, is now 41% of predicted, and her peak expiratory flow rate (PEFR) is 13% of predicted. Arterial blood gases show pH 7.37, PaO_2 69 mm Hg, and $PaCO_2$ 44 mm Hg. You start treatment with bronchodilators and corticosteroids and are considering whether the patient would be best treated in an intermediate care unit when one of your junior colleagues suggests treatment with intravenous magnesium sulfate. You are altogether uncertain about this suggestion and so offer nothing more than a polite acknowledgement, but she returns 15 minutes later with a printout of Cochrane Library review dealing with the topic.[1]

FINDING THE EVIDENCE

In this scenario, a colleague provided the relevant article from the Cochrane Library. Were you searching "asthma and magnesium," you could have found this article by entering the Cochrane Library and by typing "magnesium and asthma." You could also find it quickly in

ACP Journal Club by typing the same terms and in UpToDate by looking in their asthma section, narrowing it by magnesium and looking into "alternative agents for treatment of asthma."

Traditional Narrative and Systematic Reviews

The large number of studies addressing many clinical questions makes *review articles* an efficient way to learn about relevant *evidence*. In the same way that it is important to use rigorous methods in primary research to protect against *bias* and *random error*, it is also important to use rigorous methods when summarizing the results of several studies. Traditional literature reviews, commonly found in journals and textbooks, typically provide *narrative reviews* of a disease or condition. Traditional narrative reviews often include a discussion of 1 or more aspects of disease etiology, diagnosis, *prognosis*, or management and address a number of *background questions*, *foreground questions*, and theoretical questions.

Typically, authors of traditional reviews make little or no attempt to be systematic in their formulation of the questions they are addressing, their search for and selection of evidence, their assessment of the quality of *primary studies*, and their summary of the results of the primary studies. Medical students and clinicians looking for background information often find narrative reviews useful for obtaining a broad overview of a clinical condition (see Chapter 3, What Is the Question? and Chapter 4, Finding the Evidence).

Unfortunately, expert reviewers often make conflicting recommendations, and their advice has frequently lagged behind or has been inconsistent with the best available evidence.[2] One important reason for this phenomenon is the use of unsystematic approaches to collecting and summarizing the evidence. Indeed, in one study, self-rated expertise was inversely related to the methodologic rigor of the review.[3]

Although most *systematic reviews* focus on issues of the effect of interventions, they can also address issues of diagnosis and prognosis and even questions of how and why addressed by qualitative research studies (sometimes called *meta-synthesis*). In this chapter, although we focus on systematic reviews that address discrete patient management issues, the principles for other types of questions are similar.

Authors sometimes erroneously use the terms *systematic review* and *meta-analysis* interchangeably. We use the term *systematic review* for any summary of research that attempts to address a focused clinical question in a systematic, reproducible manner and *meta-analysis* for the quantitative synthesis that yields a single best estimate of, for instance, *treatment effect*. Most articles labeled as meta-analyses published in the biomedical literature are actually systematic reviews that statistically pool the results of 2 or more primary studies. Features distinguishing narrative reviews from systematic reviews and meta-analyses are shown in Table 14-1.[4]

During the past decade, the literature describing the optimal methods for systematic reviews has grown enormously and now includes studies that provide an empirical basis for guiding decisions about the methods used in summarizing evidence.[5,6] Here, we

TABLE 14-1

Differences Between Narrative and Systematic Reviews

Characteristic	Narrative Review	Systematic Review
Clinical question	Seldom reported, or addresses several general questions	Focused question specifying population, intervention or exposure, and outcome
Search for primary articles	Seldom reported; if reported, not comprehensive	Comprehensive search of several evidence sources
Selection of primary articles	Seldom reported; if reported, often biased sample of studies	Explicit inclusion and exclusion criteria for primary studies
Evaluation of quality of primary articles	Seldom reported; if reported, not usually systematic	Methodologic quality of primary articles is assessed
Summary of results of primary studies	Usually qualitative nonsystematic summary	Synthesis is systematic (qualitative or quantitative; if quantitative, this is often referred to as meta-analysis)

Reproduced from Cook et al.[4]

emphasize key points from the perspective of a clinician needing to make a decision about patient care.

A Roadmap for Systematic Reviews

In applying the Users' Guides, you will find it useful to have a clear understanding of the process of conducting a systematic review. Figure 14-1 demonstrates how the process begins with the definition

FIGURE 14-1

The Process of Conducting a Systematic Review

Define the question
  • Specify inclusion and exclusion criteria
        Population
        Intervention or exposure
        Outcome
        Methodology (including time, language, publication restrictions)

Conduct literature search
  • Decide on information sources: databases, experts, funding
    agencies, pharmaceutical companies, hand-searching,
    personal files, trial registries, Cochrane Database of randomized
    controlled trials, citation lists of retrieved articles
  • Identify titles and abstracts

Apply inclusion and exclusion criteria
  • Apply inclusion and exclusion criteria to titles and abstracts
  • Obtain full articles for eligible titles and abstracts
  • Apply inclusion and exclusion criteria to full articles
  • Select final eligible articles
  • Assess agreement on study selection

Create data abstraction
  • Data abstraction: participants, interventions, comparison
    interventions, study design
  • Results
  • Methodologic quality
  • Assess agreement on validity assessment

Conduct analysis
  • Determine method of generating pooled estimates across studies
  • Generate pooled estimates (if appropriate)
  • Explore heterogeneity, conduct subgroup analysis if appropriate
  • Explore possibility of publications bias

of the question, which is synonymous with specifying eligibility criteria for deciding which studies to include in a review. These criteria define the population, the *exposures* or interventions, and the outcomes of interest. Depending on the scope of their review, authors may need to decide at this stage which *outcome* measures will be crucial for clinical decision makers and ensure they summarize the evidence for each of these outcomes. A systematic review will also restrict the included studies to those that meet minimal methodologic standards. For example, systematic reviews that address a question of therapy will often include only *randomized controlled trials (RCTs)*.

Having specified their selection criteria, reviewers must conduct a comprehensive search that yields a large number of potentially relevant titles and abstracts. They then apply the selection criteria to the titles and abstracts, arriving at a smaller number of articles that they can retrieve. Once again, the reviewers apply the selection criteria, this time to the complete reports. Having completed the culling process, they assess the methodologic quality of the articles and abstract data from each study. Finally, they summarize the data, including, if appropriate, a quantitative synthesis or meta-analysis. The analysis includes an examination of differences among the included studies, an attempt to explain differences in results (exploring *heterogeneity*), a summary of the overall results, and an overall assessment of methodologic quality. Guidelines for assessing the validity of reviews and using the results correspond to this process (Table 14-2).

ARE THE RESULTS VALID?

Did the Review Explicitly Address a Sensible Clinical Question?

Consider a systematic review that pooled results from all cancer therapeutic modalities for all types of cancer to generate a single estimate of the effect on mortality. Next, consider a review that pooled the results of the effects of all doses of all antiplatelet agents

TABLE 14-2

Users' Guides for How to Use Review Articles

Are the results valid?
- Did the review include explicit and appropriate eligibility criteria?
- Was biased selection and reporting of studies unlikely?
- Were the primary studies of high methodologic quality?
- Were assessments of studies reproducible?

What are the results?
- Were the results similar from study to study?
- What are the overall results of the review?
- How precise were the results?

How can I apply the results to patient care?
- Were all patient-important outcomes considered?
- Are any postulated subgroup effects credible?
- What is the overall quality of the evidence?
- Are the benefits worth the costs and potential risks?

(including aspirin, sulfinpyrazone, dipyridamole, ticlodipine, and clopidogrel) on major thrombotic events (including myocardial infarctions, strokes, and acute arterial insufficiency in the leg) and mortality in patients with clinically manifest atherosclerosis (whether in the heart, head, or lower extremities). Finally, reflect on a review that addressed the influence of a wide range of aspirin doses to prevent thrombotic stroke in patients who had experienced a transient ischemic attack (TIA) in the carotid circulation.

Clinicians would not find the first of these reviews useful; they would conclude it is too broad. Most clinicians are uncomfortable with the second question, still considering it excessively broad. For this second question, however, a highly credible and experienced group of investigators found the question reasonable and published the results of their meta-analysis in a leading journal.[7-10] Most clinicians are comfortable with the third question, although they may express concerns about pooling across a wide range of aspirin doses.

What makes a systematic review too broad or too narrow? When deciding whether the question posed in the review is sensible, clinicians need to ask themselves whether the underlying biology is what they would more or less expect; that is, the same treatment effect across the range of patients (Table 14-3). They should ask the parallel question about the other components of the study question: Is the underlying biology such that, across the range of interventions and outcomes included, they expect more or less the same treatment effect? Clinicians can also construct a similar set of questions for other areas of clinical inquiry. For example, across the range of patients, ways of testing, and *reference* or *gold standard* for diagnosis, does one expect more or less the same *likelihood ratios* associated with studies examining a diagnostic test (see Chapter 12, Diagnostic Tests)?[11]

Clinicians reject a systematic review that pools data across all modes of cancer therapy for all types of cancer because they know that some cancer treatments are effective in certain cancers, whereas others are harmful. Combining the results of these studies would yield an estimate of effect that would be misleading for most of the interventions. Clinicians who reject the second review would argue that the biologic variation in antiplatelet agents is likely to lead to

TABLE 14-3

Were Eligibility Criteria Appropriate?

Are results likely to be similar across the range of patients included (eg, older and younger, sicker and less sick)?

Are results likely to be similar across the range of interventions or exposures studied (eg, higher dose lower dose; test interpreted by expert or nonexpert)?

Are results likely to be similar across the range of ways the outcome was measured (eg, shorter or longer follow-up)?

Did it turn out that results were indeed similar across the range of patients, interventions, and outcomes (ie, studies all showed similar results)?

important differences in treatment effect. Furthermore, they may contend that there are important differences in the biology of atherosclerosis in the vessels of the heart, head, and legs. Those who would endorse the second review would argue the similar underlying biology of antiplatelet agents—and atherosclerosis in different parts of the body—and thus anticipate a similar magnitude of treatment effects.

For the third question, most clinicians would accept that the biology of aspirin action is likely to be similar in patients whose TIA reflected right-sided or left-sided brain ischemia, in patients older than 75 years and in younger patients, in men and women, across doses, during periods of *follow-up* ranging from 1 to 5 years, and in patients with stroke who have been identified by the attending physician and those identified by a team of expert reviewers. The similar biology is likely to result in a similar magnitude of treatment effect, which explains the reviewers' comfort with combining studies of aspirin in patients who have had a TIA.

The clinician's task is to decide whether, across the range of patients, interventions or exposures, and outcomes, it is plausible that the intervention will have a similar effect. This judgment is possible only if the reviewers have provided a precise statement of what range of patients, exposures, and outcomes they decided to include; in other words, explicit eligibility criteria for their review.

In addition, reviewers must specify methodologic criteria for inclusion in their review. Generally, these should be similar to the most important *validity* criteria for primary studies (Table 14-4). Explicit eligibility criteria not only facilitate the decision regarding whether the question was sensible but also make it less likely that the authors will preferentially include studies that support their own previous conclusions.

Clinicians may legitimately ask, even within a relatively narrowly defined question, whether they can be confident that results will be similar across patients, interventions, and outcome measurement. Referring to the question of aspirin in patients with a TIA, the effect could conceivably differ in those with more or less severe underlying atherosclerosis, across aspirin doses, or during short-term and long-term follow-up. Thus, this validity criterion cannot be fully resolved

TABLE 14-4

Guides for Selecting Articles That Are Most Likely to Provide Valid Results[3]

Therapy	• Were patients randomized?
	• Was follow-up complete?
Diagnosis	• Was the patient sample representative of those with the disorder?
	• Was the diagnosis verified using credible criteria that were independent of the items of medical history, physical examination, laboratory tests, or imaging procedures under study?
Harm	• Did the investigators demonstrate similarity in all known determinants of outcome or adjust for differences in the analysis?
	• Was follow-up sufficiently complete?
Prognosis	• Was there a representative sample of patients?
	• Was follow-up sufficiently complete?

until one examines the results. Anticipating possible variability in results, reviewers should generate a priori hypotheses of features of population, intervention, outcome, and methodology that might explain such variability (Figure 14-1). As we describe in the "Results" section of this chapter, if there is large variation in results across studies that reviewers' a priori hypotheses cannot explain, our confidence in the estimates of effect is compromised.

Was the Search for Relevant Studies Detailed and Exhaustive?

Systematic reviews are at risk of presenting misleading results if they fail to secure a complete, or at least a representative, sample of the available eligible studies. To achieve this objective, reviewers search bibliographic databases, such as MEDLINE and EMBASE and the Cochrane Central Register of Controlled Trials (containing more than 450 000 RCTs), and databases of current research.[12] They check the reference lists of the articles they retrieve and seek personal contact with experts in the area. It may also be important to examine recently published abstracts presented at scientific meetings and to look at less frequently used databases, including those that summarize doctoral theses and databases of ongoing trials held by pharmaceutical companies. Unless the authors tell us what they did to locate relevant studies, it is difficult to know how likely it is that relevant studies were missed.

Reporting bias occurs in a number of forms, the most familiar of which is the failure to report or publish studies with negative results. This *publication bias* may result in misleading results of systematic reviews that fail to include unpublished studies.[13-18]

If investigators include unpublished studies in a review, they should obtain full written reports and they should use the same criteria to appraise the validity of both published and unpublished studies. There is a variety of techniques available to explore the possibility of publication bias, none of them fully satisfactory. Systematic reviews based on a number of small studies with limited total sample sizes are particularly susceptible to publication bias, especially if most or all of the studies have been sponsored by a commercial entity with a vested interest in the results. Findings that seem too good to be true may well not be true.

Another increasingly recognized form of reporting bias occurs when investigators measure a number of outcomes but report only those that favor the experimental intervention or those that favor the intervention most strongly (this is sometimes referred to as *selective outcome reporting bias*). If reviewers report that they have successfully contacted authors of primary studies who ensure full disclosure of results, concern about reporting bias decreases.

Reviewers may go even farther than simply contacting the authors of primary studies. They may recruit these investigators as collaborators in their review, and in the process, they may obtain individual patient records. Such *individual patient-data meta-analysis* can facilitate powerful analyses (addressing issues such as true *intention-to-treat* analyses, informed subgroup analyses), which may strengthen the inferences from a systematic review.

Were the Primary Studies of High Methodologic Quality?

Even if a systematic review includes only RCTs, knowing whether they were of good quality is important. Unfortunately, peer review does not guarantee the validity of published research.[19] Differences in study methods might explain important differences among the results.[20-22] For example, less rigorous studies tend to overestimate the effectiveness of therapeutic and preventive interventions.[23] Even if the results of different studies are consistent, determining their validity still is important. Consistent results are less compelling if they come from weak studies than if they come from strong studies.

Consistent results from *observational studies* putatively addressing treatment issues are particularly suspect. Physicians may systematically select patients with a good prognosis to receive therapy; and this pattern of practice may be consistent over time and geographic setting. Observational studies summarized in a systematic review,[24] for instance, have consistently shown average *relative risk reductions* in major cardiovascular events with hormone replacement therapy. The first large RCT addressing this issue found no effect of hormone replacement therapy on cardiovascular risk,[25] and the subsequent large RCT suggested possibly detrimental effect.[26-28] Hormone replacement therapy is one of many examples of misleading results of observational studies.[29]

All we have said about validity applies to the focus of this chapter: systematic reviews assessing questions of therapy. Investigators may also undertake systematic reviews of issues concerning diagnosis or prognosis. Different validity criteria (corresponding to the validity criteria of the prognosis and diagnosis chapters of this book) are appropriate for such systematic reviews.

There is no one correct way to assess the quality of studies, and clinicians should be cautious about the use of scales to assess the quality of studies.[30,31] Some reviewers use long checklists to evaluate methodologic quality, whereas others focus on 3 or 4 key aspects of the study. When considering whether to trust the results of a review, check to see whether the authors examined criteria similar to those we have presented in other chapters of this book (see Chapter 6, Therapy; Chapter 9, Harm; Chapter 12, Diagnostic Tests; and Chapter 13, Prognosis). Reviewers should apply these criteria with a relatively low threshold (such as restricting eligibility to RCTs) in selecting studies (Table 14-4) and more comprehensively (such as considering *concealment*, *blinding*, *stopping early* for benefit) in assessing the validity of the included studies (Figure 14-1).

Were Selection and Assessments of Studies Reproducible?

As we have seen, authors of review articles must decide which studies to include, how valid they are, and what data to abstract. These decisions require judgment by the reviewers and are subject to both mistakes (ie, random errors) and bias (ie, systematic errors). Having 2 or more people participate in each decision guards against errors; and if there is good agreement beyond chance between the reviewers, the clinician can have more confidence in the results of the systematic review.

USING THE GUIDE

Returning to our opening scenario, the Cochrane review you located included 7 trials enrolling patients who have asthma and present to the emergency department with an asthma attack, 5 of which addressed the investigators' designated primary outcome, hospitalization.[1] These patients were randomized to receive or not receive intravenous magnesium sulfate, on average 2 g during 20 minutes. The reviewers searched the Cochrane Airway Review Group asthma register and reference lists of all available primary studies and review articles, and they contacted authors of primary studies. It is likely they obtained all the relevant trials, although the relatively small number of small trials leaves some uncertainty regarding publication bias.

The authors of the review addressed concealment of randomization and also used the Jadad score that rates randomization, blinding, and loss to follow-up.[32] Of the 7 trials, 6 were randomized and placebo controlled and included some blinding; loss to follow-up was generally small. The seventh was quasi-randomized and described as "single blind." Of the 7 studies included, 6 were rated as strong and 1 as weak, according to the Jadad score.

Two of the review's authors decided whether potentially eligible trials met eligibility criteria, with disagreement resolved by consensus or third-party adjudication. The investigators report no measures of agreement for either the eligibility or quality rating decisions.

Both adults and children with varying severity of asthma were included, and authors planned a priori appropriate subgroup analyses based on age and severity. In addition to their primary outcome of need for admission to the hospital, they also considered pulmonary function tests (PEFR and FEV_1), vital signs (heart rate, respiratory rate, blood pressure), and adverse effects.

Overall, we conclude that the methods of the systematic review and the methodologic quality of the trials included in the systematic review were strong.

WHAT ARE THE RESULTS?

Were the Results Similar From Study to Study?

Most systematic reviews document important differences in patients, exposures, outcome measures, and research methods from study to study. As a result, the most common answer to whether eligibility criteria were appropriate—that is, whether we can expect similar results across the range of patients, interventions, and outcomes—is perhaps.

Fortunately, one can resolve this unsatisfactory situation. Having completed the review, investigators should present the results in a way that allows clinicians to check whether results proved similar from study to study. There are 4 elements to consider when deciding whether the results are sufficiently similar to warrant comfort with a single estimate of treatment effects that applies across the populations, interventions, and outcomes studied (Table 14-5). First, how similar are the study-specific estimates of the treatment effect (that is, the *point estimates*) from the individual studies? The more different they are, the more clinicians should question the decision to pool results across studies.

TABLE 14-5

Evaluating Variability in Study Results

Visual evaluation of variability

   How similar are the point estimates?

   To what extent do the confidence intervals overlap?

Statistical tests evaluating variability

   Yes-or-no tests for heterogeneity that generate a P value

   I^2 test that quantifies the variability explained by between-study differences in results

---

Second, to what extent are differences among the results of individual studies greater than you would expect by chance? Users can make an initial assessment by examining the extent to which the *confidence intervals (CIs)* overlap. The greater the overlap, the more comfortable one is with pooling results. Widely separated CIs flag the presence of important variability in results that requires explanation.

Clinicians can also look to formal statistical analyses called *tests for heterogeneity*, which address the null hypothesis that underlying effects are in fact similar across studies and the observed differences in the size of effect between studies are due to chance. When the P value associated with the test of heterogeneity is small (for instance, $P < .05$), chance becomes an unlikely explanation for the observed differences in the size of the effect.

A fourth criterion is another statistic, the I^2, which describes the percentage of the variability in effect estimates that is due to underlying differences in effect rather than chance.[33] Rough guides for the interpretation of I^2 suggest that a value of less than 20% represents minimal variability, 20% to 50% variability raises concern, and values greater than 50% represent substantial heterogeneity that raises serious concern about a single pooled estimate.

Reviewers should try to explain between-study variability in findings by examining differences in patients, interventions, outcome measurement, and methodology. Although appropriate and, indeed, necessary, this search for explanations of heterogeneity in study results may be misleading. Furthermore, how is the clinician to deal with residual heterogeneity in study results that remains unexplained? We will deal with this issue in the next section concerning the applicability of the study results.

What Are the Overall Results of the Review?

If the investigators decide that pooling results to generate a single estimate of effect is inappropriate, a systematic review will likely end with a table or tables describing results of individual studies. Often, however, reviewers present a meta-analysis with a single best estimate of effect from the weighted averages of the results of the individual studies. The weighting process depends on the sample size of the studies or, more specifically, the number of events.

You should look to the overall results of a systematic review the same way you look to the results of primary studies. In a systematic review of a therapeutic question looking at dichotomous (yes/no) outcomes, you should look for the *relative risk* (*RR*) and *relative risk reduction* or the *odds ratio* and *odds reduction* (see Chapter 7, Does Treatment Lower Risk? Understanding the Results). In systematic reviews regarding diagnosis, you should look for summary estimates of the likelihood ratios (see Chapter 12, Diagnostic Tests).

In the setting of continuous rather than *dichotomous outcomes*, investigators typically use one of 2 options to aggregate data across studies. If the outcome is measured the same way in each study (eg, percentage of improvement in FEV_1 or difference in liters in PEFR), the results from each study are averaged, taking into account each study's precision to calculate what is called a *weighted mean difference*.

Sometimes the outcome measures used in the primary studies are similar but not identical. For example, one trial might measure exercise capacity by using a treadmill; a second, a cycle ergometer; and a third, a 6-minute walk test. If the patients and the interventions are reasonably similar, estimating the average effect of the intervention on exercise capacity still might be worthwhile. One way of doing this is to standardize the measures by looking at the mean difference between treatment and control and dividing this by the standard deviation.[34] The *effect size* that results from this calculation provides a pooled estimate of the treatment effect expressed in standard deviation units (eg, an effect size of one-half means that the average effect of treatment across studies is one-half of a standard deviation unit).

You may find it difficult to interpret the clinical importance of an effect size. Effect sizes of approximately 0.2 SD represent small effects; 0.5 SD, moderate; and 0.8, large.[35] Reviewers may help you interpret the results by translating the summary effect size back into natural units.[36] For instance, clinicians may have become familiar with the significance of differences in walk test scores in patients with chronic lung disease. Investigators can then convert the effect size of a treatment on a number of measures of functional status (eg, the walk test and stair climbing) back into differences in walk test scores.[37]

How Precise Were the Results?

In the same way that it is possible to estimate the average effect across studies, it is possible to estimate a CI around that estimate; that is, a range of values with a specified *probability* (typically 95%) of including the true effect (see Chapter 8, Confidence Intervals).

USING THE GUIDE

Returning to our opening scenario, the primary outcome, admission to the hospital, showed a trend in favor of magnesium sulfate that just reaches the threshold for *statistical significance* (RR, 0.70; 95% CI, 0.51-0.98). The results, however, are variable between studies (Figure 14-2) (the *P* value for the test of heterogeneity = .04, and the I^2 is 56%). In the severe asthma group, in contrast, the pooled difference between magnesium and *placebo* was clearly statistically significant and important (RR, 0.59; 95% CI, 0.43-0.80) and the results more consistent across studies (Figure 14-2). Four studies that enrolled patients with severe asthma included a total of 70 patients who received magnesium sulfate and 63 who received placebo; there were 56 admissions among placebo patients and 34 among active treatment patients (Figure 14-2). There were no differences in vital signs or measured adverse effects, although the authors indicate that an insufficient number of studies were available to draw firm conclusions about adverse effects and adverse events.

FIGURE 14-2

Results of Randomized Trials of Magnesium Sulphate in Asthmatic Patients Presenting to the Emergency Department

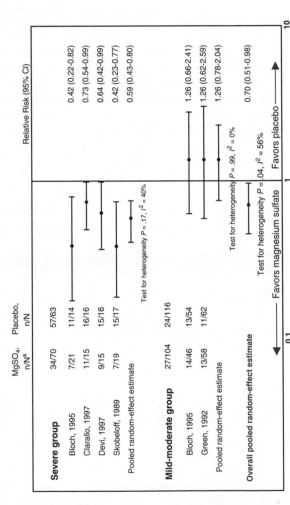

	MgSO$_4$, n/N[a]	Placebo, n/N	Relative Risk (95% CI)
Severe group	34/70	57/63	
Bloch, 1995	7/21	11/14	0.42 (0.22-0.82)
Ciarallo, 1997	11/15	16/16	0.73 (0.54-0.99)
Devi, 1997	9/15	15/16	0.64 (0.42-0.99)
Skobeloff, 1989	7/19	15/17	0.42 (0.23-0.77)
Pooled random-effect estimate			0.59 (0.43-0.80)

Test for heterogeneity $P = .17$, $I^2 = 40\%$

Mild-moderate group	27/104	24/116	
Bloch, 1995	14/46	13/54	1.26 (0.66-2.41)
Green, 1992	13/58	11/62	1.26 (0.62-2.59)
Pooled random-effect estimate			1.26 (0.78-2.04)

Test for heterogeneity $P = .99$, $I^2 = 0\%$

Overall pooled random-effect estimate			0.70 (0.51-0.98)

Test for heterogeneity $P = .04$, $I^2 = 56\%$

Favors magnesium sulfate ← → Favors placebo

[a]n/N = Hospitalizations/total sample.

How Can I Apply the Results to Patient Care?

Were All Patient-Important Outcomes Considered?

Although it is a good idea to look for focused systematic review articles because they are more likely to provide accurate results, this does not mean that you should ignore outcomes that are not included in a review. For example, the potential benefits of hormone replacement therapy include a reduced risk of fractures and a reduced risk of colon cancer, and potential downsides include an increased risk of breast cancer and, surprisingly, possibly of adverse cardiovascular outcomes. Focused reviews of the evidence are more likely to provide accurate results of the impact of hormone replacement therapy on each of these 4 outcomes, but a clinical decision requires considering all of them. The best systematic review is a series of such reviews, one for each *patient-important outcome*.

Systematic reviews frequently do not report the adverse effects of therapy. One reason is that the individual studies often measure these adverse effects either in different ways or not at all, making pooling, or even effective summarization, difficult. Costs are an additional outcome that you will often find absent from systematic reviews.

Are Any Postulated Subgroup Effects Credible?

The extent to which one finds subgroup analyses credible is often pivotal in interpreting the results of systematic reviews. Even if the true underlying effect is identical in each of a set of studies, chance will ensure that the observed results differ (see Chapter 5, Why Study Results Mislead: Bias and Random Error). As a result, systematic reviews risk capitalizing on the play of chance. Perhaps the studies with sicker patients happened, by chance, to be those with the larger treatment effects. The reviewer may erroneously conclude that the treatment is more effective in sicker patients. The more subgroup analyses the reviewer undertakes, the greater the risk of a spurious conclusion.

The clinician can apply a number of criteria to distinguish subgroup analyses that are credible from those that are not (see Table 14-6). If

TABLE 14-6

Guidelines for Deciding Whether Apparent Differences in Subgroup Response Are Real

- Did the hypothesis precede rather than follow the analysis?
- Was the subgroup difference one of a small number of hypothesized effects tested?
- Is the subgroup difference suggested by comparisons within rather than between studies?
- Is the magnitude of the subgroup difference large?
- Is the subgroup difference consistent across studies?
- Was the subgroup difference statistically significant?
- Does external evidence support the hypothesized subgroup difference?

these criteria are not met, the results of a subgroup analysis are less likely to be credible and you should assume that the overall effect across all patients and all treatments, rather than the subgroup effect, applies to the patient at hand and to the treatment under consideration.

What are clinicians to do if subgroup analyses fail to provide an adequate explanation for unexplained heterogeneity in study results? Although a number of reasonable possibilities exist, including not to pool findings at all, we suggest that, pending further trials that may explain the differences, clinicians use a summary measure from all of the best available studies for the best estimate of the effect of the intervention or exposure.[38-40]

USING THE GUIDE

Your confidence in the benefit of magnesium depends on the extent to which you find the subgroup analysis focusing on severely ill patients credible. Applying the 7 criteria, we find that the investigators generated the hypothesis before they began the analysis, and it was one of only 2 subgroup hypotheses they explored. Comparisons are based on between- and, in one case, within-study comparisons (Bloch; Figure 14-2). The magnitude of the difference in effect between the severe and mild or moderate asthma is large (RRs of 0.59 and 1.26), and the difference is reasonably consistent across studies (you observe an I^2 of 40%, suggesting appreciable residual variability in results in the studies of severe patients) and is unlikely to occur by chance (P = .006) (Figure 14-2). The plausibility is less certain, but because severe asthma was usually described as a condition unresponsive to initial b-agonist treatment, one may speculate that persistent bronchospasm was required to demonstrate an effect of magnesium. Thus, the postulated subgroup effect that magnesium is effective in severe but not mild to moderate asthma meets 4 criteria completely and 3 partially. You conclude that you are ready to believe in the subgroup effect.

What Is the Overall Quality of the Evidence?

For systematic reviews that focus on alternative patient management strategies—in most instances, treatment decisions for individual patients—it may be helpful to consider the overall quality of the evidence for each patient-important outcome for each subgroup of patients (if one finds 1 or more subgroup analyses credible). An international group of clinician-methodologists and guideline developers—the GRADE Working Group—have suggested a framework for making this assessment.[41] The GRADE system provides a definition of quality of evidence: the extent to which we can be confident in the estimates of intervention effects.

In this 4-category rating system (high, moderate, low, and very low), observational studies provide only low quality of evidence unless the magnitude of effect is large (eg, hip replacement in patients with severe hip osteoarthritis). RCTs start as high-quality evidence, but a number of concerns may lead us to lower our assessment of the quality of the evidence (Table 14-7). Observational studies begin as low quality but, if the magnitude of the effect is large enough, can move up to moderate or even high quality. Some applications of this approach (eg, UpToDate) combine the 2 lowest categories of evidence, low quality and very low quality, into a single category and report their recommendations accordingly.

Are the Benefits Worth the Costs and Potential Risks?

Finally, either explicitly or implicitly, the clinician and patient must weigh the expected benefits against the costs and potential *risks* (see Chapter 15, How to Use a Patient Management Recommendation). A valid set of systematic reviews comparing the effect of alternative management strategies on all patient-important outcomes provides the best possible basis for decision making, but clinicians must still consider the results in the context of patients' *values and preferences* and in the context of your health care system's ability to deliver (see Chapter 15, How to Use a Patient Management Recommendation).

TABLE 14-7

Simplified GRADE Rating of Quality of Evidence

Randomized trials start high but move down because:

- Of poor design and implementation
- Of imprecision (wide confidence intervals)
- Of inconsistent results (variability in effect)
- Of high likelihood of publication bias

Observational studies start low but can move up because of:

- Large treatment effect

Abbreviation: GRADE, grades of recommendation, assessment, development, and evaluation.

USING THE GUIDE

The available data come from RCTs of patients with severe asthma focusing on a patient-important outcome (admission to the hospital), including methodologically strong studies, with reasonably narrow CIs, reasonably consistent results (Figure 14-2), and no strong suggestion of publication bias. On this basis, you rate the evidence as high quality. You are left, however, with 1 nagging doubt: the total number of patients with asthma is only 133 and the total number of events only 100. The authors examined adverse effects but, consistent with studies of magnesium for other conditions, they found no important adverse effects.

CLINICAL RESOLUTION

You have decided (despite the nagging doubt about the small number of patients included in the studies) that you have high-quality evidence of a large effect of magnesium in reducing the need for hospitalization in patients with asthma. You therefore administer 2 g of magnesium sulfate intravenously, in addition to bronchodilators and corticosteroids. Three hours later, the patient is feeling a little better, and you admit her to a well-monitored unit. During the next 48 hours, the patient improves and is discharged home on the third hospital day, with the strongest possible counsel to find a new home for her cat.

References

1. Rowe BH, Bretzlaff JA, Bourdon C, Bota GW, Camargo CA Jr. Magnesium sulfate for treating exacerbations of acute asthma in emergency department. Cochrane Database Syst Rev. 2000;(1): CD 001490.

2. Antman EM, Lau J, Kupelnick B, Mosteller F, Chalmers TC. A comparison of results of meta-analyses of randomized control trials and recommendations of clinical experts: treatments for myocardial infarction. *JAMA*. 1992;268(2):240-248.

3. Oxman AD, Guyatt GH. The science of reviewing research. *Ann N Y Acad Sci*. 1993;703:125-133; discussion 133-124.

4. Cook DJ, Mulrow CD, Haynes RB. Systematic reviews: synthesis of best evidence for clinical decisions. *Ann Intern Med*. 1997;126(5):376-380.

5. Higgins JPGS, ed. Cochrane handbook for systematic review of interventions 425 (updated May 2005). Chichester, UK: John Wiley & Sons, Ltd: Cochrane Library; 2005; issue 3.

6. Systematic Reviews in Health Care: Meta-Analysis in Context. 2nd ed. London, England: BMJ Books; 2000.

7. Antiplatelet Trialists' Collaboration. Collaborative overview of randomised trials of antiplatelet therapy, I: prevention of death, myocardial infarction, and stroke by prolonged antiplatelet therapy in various categories of patients. BMJ. 1994;308(6921):81-106.

8. Antiplatelet Trialists' Collaboration. Collaborative overview of randomised trials of antiplatelet therapy, II: maintenance of vascular graft or arterial patency by antiplatelet therapy. BMJ. 1994;308(6922):159-168.

9. Antiplatelet Trialists' Collaboration. Collaborative overview of randomised trials of antiplatelet therapy, III: reduction in venous thrombosis and pulmonary embolism by antiplatelet prophylaxis among surgical and medical patients. BMJ. 1994;308(6923):235-246.

10. Antithrombotic Trialists' Collaboration. Collaborative meta-analysis of randomised trials of antiplatelet therapy for prevention of death, myocardial infarction, and stroke in high risk patients. *BMJ*. 2002;324(7329):71-86.

11. Irwig L, Tosteson AN, Gatsonis C, et al. Guidelines for meta-analyses evaluating diagnostic tests. *Ann Intern Med*. 1994;120(8):667-676.

12. The *meta*Register of Controlled Trials (*m*RCT). Current controlled trials. http://www.controlled-trials.com. Accessed March 20, 2008.

13. Dickersin K. The existence of publication bias and risk factors for its occurrence. *JAMA*. 1990;263(10):1385-1389.

14. Dickersin K, Min YI, Meinert CL. Factors influencing publication of research results: follow-up of applications submitted to two institutional review boards. *JAMA*. 1992;267(3):374-378.

15. Dickersin K. How important is publication bias? a synthesis of available data. *AIDS Educ Prev*. 1997;9(1 suppl):15-21.

16. Stern JM, Simes RJ. Publication bias: evidence of delayed publication in a cohort study of clinical research projects. *BMJ*. 1997;315(7109):640-645.

17. Ioannidis JP. Effect of the statistical significance of results on the time to completion and publication of randomized efficacy trials. *JAMA*. 1998;279(4):281-286.

18. Eysenbach G. Tackling publication bias and selective reporting in health informatics research: register your eHealth trials in the International eHealth Studies Registry. *J Med Internet Res*. 2004;6(3):e35.

19. Williamson JW, Goldschmidt PG, Colton T. The quality of medical literature: an analysis of validation assessments. In: Bailar JC, Mosteller F. *Medical Uses of Statistics*. 2nd ed. Waltham, MA: NEJM Books; 1992.

20. Horwitz RI. Complexity and contradiction in clinical trial research. *Am J Med*. 1987;82(3):498-510.

21. Detsky AS, Naylor CD, O'Rourke K, McGeer AJ, L'Abbe KA. Incorporating variations in the quality of individual randomized trials into meta-analysis. *J Clin Epidemiol*. 1992;45(3):255-265.

22. Moher D, Pham B, Jones A, et al. Does quality of reports of randomised trials affect estimates of intervention efficacy reported in meta-analyses? *Lancet*. 1998;352(9128):609-613.

23. Kunz R, Oxman AD. The unpredictability paradox: review of empirical comparisons of randomised and non-randomised clinical trials. *BMJ*. 1998;317(7167):1185-1190.

24. Stampfer MJ, Colditz GA. Estrogen replacement therapy and coronary heart disease: a quantitative assessment of the epidemiologic evidence. *Prev Med*. 1991;20(1):47-63.

25. Hulley S, Grady D, Bush T, et al. Randomized trial of estrogen plus progestin for secondary prevention of coronary heart disease in postmenopausal women: Heart and Estrogen/progestin Replacement Study (HERS) Research Group. *JAMA*. 1998;280(7):605-613.

26. Nelson HD, Humphrey LL, Nygren P, Teutsch SM, Allan JD. Postmenopausal hormone replacement therapy: scientific review. *JAMA*. 2002;288(7):872-881.

27. Manson JE, Hsia J, Johnson KC, et al. Estrogen plus progestin and the risk of coronary heart disease. *N Engl J Med*. 2003;349(6):523-534.

28. Anderson GL, Limacher M, Assaf AR, et al. Effects of conjugated equine estrogen in postmenopausal women with hysterectomy: the Women's Health Initiative randomized controlled trial. *JAMA*. 2004;291(14):1701-1712.

29. Lacchetti C, Ioannidis J, Guyatt G. Surprising results of randomized trials. Chapter 9.2. In: Guyatt G, Rennie D, eds. *Users' Guides to the Medical Literature: A Manual for Evidence-Based Clinical Practice*, 2nd ed. New York, NY: McGraw-Hill, 2008.

30. Moher D, Jadad AR, Nichol G, Penman M, Tugwell P, Walsh S. Assessing the quality of randomized controlled trials: an annotated bibliography of scales and checklists. *Control Clin Trials*. 1995;16(1):62-73.

31. Juni P, Witschi A, Bloch R, Egger M. The hazards of scoring the quality of clinical trials for meta-analysis. *JAMA*. 1999;282(11):1054-1060.

32. Jadad AR, Moore RA, Carroll D, et al. Assessing the quality of reports of randomized clinical trials: is blinding necessary? *Control Clin Trials*. 1996;17(1):1-12.

33. Higgins JP, Thompson SG, Deeks JJ, Altman DG. Measuring inconsistency in meta-analyses. BMJ. 2003;327(7414):557-560.

34. Rosenthal R. Meta-analytic Procedures for Social Research. 2nd ed. Newbury Park, CA: Sage Publications; 1991.

35. Cohen J. *Statistical Power Analysis for the Behavioral Sciences*. 2nd ed. Hillsdale, NJ: Lawrence Earlbaum Associates; 1988.

36. Smith K, Cook D, Guyatt GH, Madhavan J, Oxman AD. Respiratory muscle training in chronic airflow limitation: a meta-analysis. *Am Rev Respir Dis*. 1992;145(3):533-539.

37. Lacasse Y, Wong E, Guyatt GH, King D, Cook DJ, Goldstein RS. Meta-analysis of respiratory rehabilitation in chronic obstructive pulmonary disease. *Lancet.* 1996;348(9035):1115-1119.

38. Peto R. Why do we need systematic overviews of randomized trials? *Stat Med*. 1987;6(3):233-244.

39. Oxman AD, Guyatt GH. A consumer's guide to subgroup analyses. *Ann Intern Med*. 1992;116(1):78-84.

40. Yusuf S, Wittes J, Probstfield J, Tyroler HA. Analysis and interpretation of treatment effects in subgroups of patients in randomized clinical trials. *JAMA*. 1991;266(1):93-98.

41. Guyatt G, Gutterman D, Baumann MH, et al. Grading strength of recommendations and quality of evidence in clinical guidelines: report from an American College of Chest Physicians Task Force. *Chest*. 2006;129(1):174-181.

How to Use a Patient Management Recommendation

Gordon Guyatt, Kameshwar Prasad,
Holger Schunemann, Roman Jaeschke,
and Deborah J. Cook

IN THIS CHAPTER:

Do the Authors Indicate the Strength of Their Recommendations?

Clinical Resolution

CLINICAL SCENARIO

Warfarin in Atrial Fibrillation: Is It the Best Choice for This Patient?

You are a primary care practitioner considering the possibility of warfarin therapy in a 76-year-old woman with congestive heart failure and chronic atrial fibrillation who has just entered your practice. Aspirin is the only antithrombotic agent that the patient has received during the 10 years she has had atrial fibrillation. Her other medical problems include hypertension, which she has had since sometime in her fifth decade and for which she has been taking hydrochlorothiazide and metoprolol, which also serves to control her heart rate. The patient does not have valvular disease, diabetes, or other comorbidity, and she does not smoke.

You are concerned that the patient might have difficulties complying with regular monitoring of her international normalized ratio and that warfarin would present a risk of serious gastrointestinal bleeding that would prove to be greater than its benefit in terms of stroke prevention. During discussion, you learn that she places a high value on avoiding a stroke and a somewhat lower value on avoiding a major bleeding episode and would accept the inconvenience associated with monitoring anticoagulant therapy.

You consider this a good opportunity to review the *evidence* and so make no change to the patient's medication regimen today, but you make a note to yourself to reconsider when she returns for her regular visit in a month's time.

Finding the Evidence

Reviewing the voluminous original literature relating to anticoagulant therapy in atrial fibrillation would take far more time than you have available, but you hope to find an evidence-based recommendation to guide you. You decide to search for 2 sources of such a recommendation: a *practice guideline* and a *decision analysis*.

You bring up your Web browser and go to your favorite search engine, http://www.Google.com. Entering the term "practice guidelines," you see that one of the first items on the results list is "National Guideline Clearinghouse," at http://www.guideline.gov. You note that the site contains "evidence-based clinical practice guidelines" and is an initiative of the US Agency for Health Care Research and Quality, formerly known as the Agency for Health Care Policy and Research, which supports the production of reputable evidence summaries.

You observe on the left side of the screen that you can "browse" the site, and after clicking on this option, you find the first page includes a number of directly relevant guidelines. You choose the most recent of these, revised in September 2004: "Antithrombotic Therapy in Atrial Fibrillation: Seventh ACCP Consensus Conference on Antithrombotic and Thrombolytic Therapy," from the American College of Chest Physicians. Clicking on the guideline, you find that it has been published in the peer-reviewed literature,[1] and clicking on Go to Complete Summary, you print the text that appears. You also send an e-mail message to the hospital librarian, asking for a copy of the published article.

Returning to http://www.Google.com, you enter the phrase "atrial fibrillation decision analysis" in the search text box, and then, clicking on the first item, you find a decision analysis published in *Lancet*[2] that appears highly suitable and that you also order from the library.

Treatment Recommendations Require a Structured Process

Each day, clinicians face dozens of patient management decisions. These decisions involve weighing benefits against harms, burden, and cost—which we will refer to as downsides of treatment—and recommending or instituting a course of action consistent with the patient's best interest. Each decision involves a consideration of the relevant evidence and a weighing of the likely benefits and downsides in light of the patient's values and preferences. When considering choices, clinicians may benefit from structured enumeration of the options and outcomes, systematic review of the evidence regarding the relationship between options and outcomes, and recommendations regarding the best choices. This chapter explores the process of developing recommendations, suggests how that process may be conducted systematically, and provides a guide for differentiating recommendations that are more rigorous (and thus more trustworthy) from those that are less rigorous (and thus are more likely to be misleading).

Failure to follow a rigorous process may lead to variability in recommendations. For example, various recommendations emerged from different meta-analyses of selective decontamination of the gut using antibiotic prophylaxis for pneumonia in critically ill patients despite similar results. The recommendations varied from suggesting implementation, to equivocation, to rejecting implementation.[3-6] Historically, expert recommendations regarding therapy for patients with myocardial infarction have often been contradictory, lagged behind the evidence, and been inconsistent with the evidence.[7]

This chapter outlines the steps involved in developing a recommendation and introduces 2 formal processes that experts and authoritative bodies use in developing recommendations: clinical practice guidelines and decision analysis. We will offer criteria for deciding when the process is done well and when it is done poorly, along with a hierarchy of treatment recommendations that clinicians may find useful.

DEVELOPING RECOMMENDATIONS

Figure 15-1 presents the steps involved in developing a recommendation, along with formal strategies for doing so. The first step in clinical decision making is to define the decision. This involves specifying the

FIGURE 15-1

A Schematic View of the Process of Developing a Treatment Recommendation

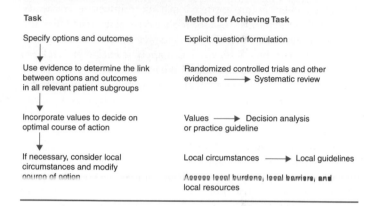

Task	Method for Achieving Task
Specify options and outcomes	Explicit question formulation
Use evidence to determine the link between options and outcomes in all relevant patient subgroups	Randomized controlled trials and other evidence ⟶ Systematic review
Incorporate values to decide on optimal course of action	Values ⟶ Decision analysis or practice guideline
If necessary, consider local circumstances and modify course of action	Local circumstances ⟶ Local guidelines Assess local burdens, local barriers, and local resources

alternative courses of action and the possible outcomes. Often, treatments are designed to delay or prevent an adverse outcome such as stroke, death, or myocardial infarction. As usual, we will refer to the outcomes that treatment is designed to prevent as *target outcomes*. Treatments are associated with their own adverse outcomes: adverse effects, toxicity, and inconvenience. In addition, new treatments may markedly increase or decrease costs. Ideally, the formulation of the question will be comprehensive, including all reasonable alternatives and all important beneficial and adverse outcomes.

In patients such as the woman with nonvalvular atrial fibrillation described in the opening scenario, options for stroke prophylaxis include no intervention, giving aspirin, or administering anticoagulant therapy with warfarin. Outcomes include minor and major embolic stroke, intracranial hemorrhage, gastrointestinal hemorrhage, minor bleeding, the inconvenience associated with taking and monitoring medication, and costs to the patient, the health care system, and society.

Having identified the options and outcomes, decision makers must evaluate the links between the two. What will the alternative management strategies yield in terms of benefit and harm?[7,8] How are potential benefits and downsides likely to vary in different groups of patients?[8,9] Once these questions are answered, making treatment recommendations involves judgments about the relative desirability or undesirability of possible outcomes, issues of values and preferences.

We will now discuss how one can apply scientific principles to the identification, selection, and summarization of evidence and to the valuing of outcomes that are involved in creating practice guidelines and decision analyses.

Practice Guidelines

Practice guidelines, systematically developed statements to assist practitioner and patient decisions about appropriate health care for specific clinical circumstances,[10] provide an alternative structure for integrating evidence and applying values to reach treatment recommendations.[1,11-16] Instead of precise quantitation, practice guidelines rely on the consensus of a group of decision makers who consider the evidence and decide on its implications. Guideline developers' mandate may be to adduce recommendations for a large part of the world, a country, a region, a city, a hospital, or a clinic. Depending on whether the country is the Philippines or the United States, whether the region is urban or rural, whether the institution is a large teaching hospital or a small community hospital, and whether the clinic serves a poor community or an affluent one, guidelines based on the same evidence may differ. For example, guideline developers may recommend against the administration of warfarin to even high-risk patients with atrial fibrillation if their recommendation is designed for rural parts of countries without resources to monitor anticoagulant intensity.

Decision Analysis

Rigorous decision analysis provides a formal structure for integrating the evidence about the beneficial and harmful effects of treatment options with the values or preferences associated with those beneficial and harmful effects. Decision analysis applies explicit, quantitative methods to analyze decisions under conditions of uncertainty; it allows clinicians to compare the expected consequences of pursuing different strategies. The process of decision analysis makes fully explicit all of the elements of the decision, so that they are open for debate and modification.[17-19]

Although clinicians may undertake such analyses to inform a decision for an individual patient (Should I recommend warfarin to this 76-year-old woman with atrial fibrillation?), most decision analyses help inform clinical policy[20] (Should I routinely recommend warfarin to patients in my practice with atrial fibrillation?).

Most clinical decision analyses are built as decision trees, and authors will usually include 1 or more diagrams showing the structure of the decision trees used for the analysis. Reviewing such diagrams will help you understand the model. Figure 15-2 shows a diagram of a simplified decision tree for the atrial fibrillation problem presented at the beginning of this chapter. The clinician has 3 options for such patients: to offer no prophylaxis, recommend aspirin, or recommend warfarin. Regardless of the choice, patients may or may not develop embolic events and, in particular, stroke. Prophylaxis decreases the chance of embolism but can cause bleeding in some patients. This simplified model excludes a number of important consequences, including the inconvenience of warfarin monitoring and the unpleasantness of minor bleeding.

As seen in Figure 15-2, decision trees are displayed graphically, oriented from left to right, with the decision to be analyzed on the left, the compared strategies in the center, and the clinical outcomes on the right. The decision is represented by a square, termed a "decision node." The lines emanating from the decision node represent the clinical strategies under consideration. Circles, called "chance nodes," symbolize chance events, and triangles or rectangles identify outcome states (Figure 15-2). When a decision analysis includes costs among the outcomes, it becomes an economic analysis and summarizes tradeoffs between health changes and resource expenditure.[21,22]

Once a decision analyst has constructed the tree, he or she must generate quantitative estimates of the likelihood of events,

FIGURE 15-2

Simplified Decision Tree for a Patient With Atrial Fibrillation

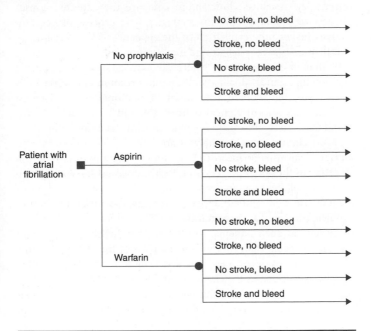

or *probabilities*. As usual for any event, probabilities may range from 0 (impossible) to 1.0 or 100% (certainty). The analyst must assign probabilities to each branch emanating from a chance node, and for each chance node, the sum of probabilities must add up to 1.0.

For example, returning to Figure 15-2, consider the no-prophylaxis strategy (the upper branch emanating from the decision node). This arm has 1 chance node at which 4 possible events could occur (the 4 possible combinations arising from bleeding or not bleeding and from having a stroke or not having a stroke). Figure 15-3 depicts the probabilities associated with one arm of the decision, the no-prophylaxis strategy (generated by assuming a 1% chance of bleeding and a 10% probability of stroke, with the 2 events being independent): Patients given no prophylaxis would have a 0.1% chance (a probability of .001) of bleeding and having a stroke, a 0.9%

FIGURE 15-3

Decision Tree With Probabilities: No-Prophylaxis Option

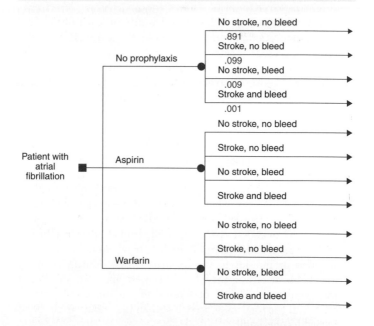

chance (a probability of .009) of bleeding and not having a stroke, a 9.9% chance (a probability of .099) of not bleeding but having a stroke, and an 89.1% chance (a probability of .891) of not bleeding and not having a stroke.

The decision analyst would generate similar probabilities for the other 2 branches. Presumably, the aspirin branch would have a higher risk of bleeding and a lower risk of stroke. The warfarin branch would have the highest risk of bleeding and the lowest risk of stroke.

These probabilities would not suggest a clear course of action, because the alternative with the lowest risk of bleeding has the highest risk of stroke, and vice versa. Thus, the right choice would depend on the relative value or utility one placed on bleeding and stroke.

Decision analysts typically place a utility on each of the final possible outcomes that varies from 0 (death) to 1.0 (full health). Figure 15-4 presents one possible set of utilities associated with the 4 outcomes and applied to the no-prophylaxis arm of the decision tree: 1.0 for no stroke or bleeding, 0.8 for no stroke and bleeding, 0.5 for stroke but no bleeding, and 0.4 for stroke and bleeding.

The final step in the decision analysis is to calculate the total expected value—the sum of the probabilities and utilities associated with each outcome—for each possible course of action. Given the particular set of probabilities and utilities we have presented, the value of the no-prophylaxis branch would be $(.891 \times 1.0) + (.009 \times .8) + (.099 \times .5) + (.001 \times .4)$, or .948. Depending on the probabilities attached to the aspirin and warfarin branches, they would be judged superior or inferior to the no-prophylaxis branch. If the total value of each of these branches were greater than .948, they would be judged preferable to the no-prophylaxis branch; if the total value were less than .948, they would be judged less desirable.

FIGURE 15-4

Decision Tree With Probabilities and Utilities Included in the No-Prophylaxis Arm of the Tree

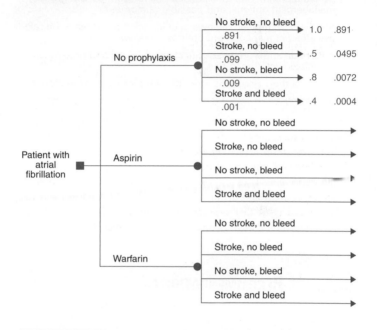

The model presented in Figures 15-2 to 15-4 is oversimplified in a number of ways, among which are its omission of the period of events and the possibility of a patient experiencing multiple events. Decision analysts can make use of software programs that model what might happen to a hypothetical cohort of patients during a series of time cycles (say, periods of 1 year's duration). The model allows for the possibility that patients might move from one health state to another. For instance, one unfortunate patient may have a mild stroke in one cycle, continue with minimal functional limitation for a number of cycles, experience a gastrointestinal bleeding

TABLE 15-1

Users' Guides for the Validity of Treatment Recommendations

- Do the recommendations consider all relevant patient groups, management options, and possible outcomes?
- Are there systematic reviews of evidence that estimate the relative effect of management options on relevant outcomes?
- Is there an appropriate specification of values and preferences associated with outcomes?
- Do the authors grade the strength of their recommendations?

episode in a subsequent cycle, and finally experience a major stroke. These *multistate transition models* or *Markov models* permit more sophisticated and true-to-life depictions.

Both decision analyses and practice guidelines can be methodologically strong or weak and thus may yield either valid or invalid recommendations. In Table 15-1, we offer 4 guidelines to assess the validity of a treatment recommendation, one for each step depicted in Figure 15-1.

ASSESSING RECOMMENDATIONS

Do the Recommendations Consider All Relevant Patient Groups, Management Options, and Possible Outcomes?

Regardless of whether recommendations apply to diagnosis, prevention, therapy, or rehabilitation, they should specify all relevant patient groups, the interventions of interest, and sensible alternative practices (Table 15-2).

For example, a guideline based on a careful systematic literature review[23] offered recommendations for medical therapeutic options for preventing strokes.[24] Although the authors mention carotid endarterectomy as an alternative in their practice guidelines, the procedure is not included in the

TABLE 15-2

Did the Recommendations Consider All Patient Groups, Management Options, and Outcomes?

Did the recommendation consider all relevant patient groups?

- Low risk and high risk
- More and less susceptible to adverse effects

Did the recommendation consider all relevant management options?

- Surgical and medical
- No-treatment option

Did the recommendation consider all patient-important outcomes?

- Morbidity and mortality
- Quality of life
- Toxicity and adverse effects
- Inconvenience
- Psychological burden
- Cost to the patient or to society

recommendations themselves. These guidelines would have been more useful if medical management for transient ischemic attacks had been placed in the context of this surgical procedure, which is effective in the hands of surgeons, with low complication rates.[25]

Treatment recommendations often vary for different subgroups of patients. In particular, those at lower risk of target outcomes that treatment is designed to prevent are less likely to benefit from therapy than those who are at higher risk. The appropriateness of lipid-lowering therapy, for instance, depends very much on the presence of risk factors such as family history, hypertension, and smoking that determine a patient's risk of adverse cardiovascular events.[26] Recommendations may also differ according to patients' susceptibility to adverse events. For our patient with atrial fibrillation, for instance, we must consider her likelihood of a traumatic fall.

Recommendations must consider not only all relevant patient groups and management options but also all important consequences of the options. Evidence concerning the effects on morbidity, mortality, and quality of life is relevant to patients, and efficient use of resources dictates attention to costs. If recommendations consider costs, regardless of whether authors use the perspective of patients, insurers, or the health care system or consider broader issues such as the consequences of time lost from work, they can further affect the conclusions.

In a decision analysis concerning anticoagulant therapy for patients with dilated cardiomyopathy,[27] the authors' decision model included all of the clinical events of interest to patients (stroke, other emboli, hemorrhage, etc). The analysts measured outcomes with "quality-adjusted life expectancy," a measure that combines information about both the quantity and the quality of life. This metric fits the clinical decision well, for one can expect that warfarin might affect both the quantity and quality of life.

Are There Systematic Reviews of Evidence That Estimate the Relative Effect of Management Options on Relevant Outcomes?

Having specified options and outcomes, decision makers must then estimate the relative effect of the management options on the occurrence of each outcome. In effect, decision makers have a series of specific questions. Consider hormone replacement therapy, in which the outcomes include the incidence of hip fracture, breast cancer, endometrial cancer, myocardial infarction, stroke, and dementia, as well as quality of life. For each of these outcomes, decisions makers must have access to, or conduct, a systematic review of the evidence. Chapter 14, Summarizing the Evidence, provides Users' Guides for deciding how likely it is that collection and summarization of the evidence are free from *bias*.

Although the authors of a systematic review may reasonably abandon their project if there are no high-quality studies to summarize, those making recommendations do not have this luxury. For important but ethically, technically, or economically difficult questions, high-quality evidence may never become available. Because recommendations must deal with the best (often low-quality) evidence available, they may need to consider a variety of studies (published and unpublished). Because the quality of the evidence in support of the recommendations can vary widely, even when grounded in rigorous collection and summarization of evidence, recommendations will usually be weak recommendations if the quality of the evidence is low. The guideline developers' systematic review must summarize the quality of the evidence on which they base their recommendations.

Is There an Appropriate Specification of Values and Preferences Associated With Outcomes?

Linking treatment options with outcomes is largely a question of fact and a matter of science. Assigning preferences to outcomes is a matter of values. Consider, for example, the relative importance of small incremental risks of developing breast cancer and possibly cardiovascular disease compared with decrease in perimenopausal hot flashes. Perimenopausal women considering hormone replacement therapy must consider these tradeoffs. Consequently, it is important that authors of guidelines or decision analyses report the principal sources of such judgments and the method of seeking consensus.

Clinicians should look for information about who was involved in assigning values to outcomes or who, by influencing recommendations, was implicitly involved in assigning values. Guideline panels are often populated largely or exclusively by clinical experts. Such expert panels may be subject to intellectual, territorial, and financial biases. Although the optimal composition of a guideline panel remains uncertain, it may be that the greater participation by methodologists, frontline clinicians, and members of the general public would lead to guidelines more in keeping with the public interest. There is no composition, however, than ensures that recommendations will be consistent with the values and preferences of your patients. As a result, for recommendations in which preferences are crucial, guidelines should state the underlying value judgments on which they are based.[28-30]

> For instance, 2 chapters of the 2004 American College of Chest Physicians antithrombotic guidelines made conflicting recommendations on the basis of the same evidence. A large, well-conducted, *randomized controlled trial* (*RCT*) that included patients with cerebrovascular disease and peripheral vascular disease demonstrated a small—some might say marginal—benefit of clopidogrel over aspirin in decreasing vascular events.[31] The stroke chapter authors, in explaining their recommendation, commented on the underlying values and preferences: "This recommendation to use clopidogrel over aspirin places a relatively high value on a small absolute risk reduction in stroke rates, and a relatively low value on minimizing drug expenditures."[32] The authors of the peripheral vascular disease chapter, as a result of differing values and preferences, recommended aspirin over clopidogrel: "This recommendation places a relatively high value on avoiding large expenditures to achieve small reductions in vascular events."[33] Unfortunately, such explicit statements are, by far, the exception rather than the rule.

Clinicians using a decision analysis will not face the huge problem of implicit and hidden value judgments that affect practice guidelines. The reason, as Figure 15-4 demonstrates, is that decision analysis requires explicit and quantitative specification of values. These values, expressed as utilities, represent measurements of the value to the decision maker of the various outcomes of the decision. Several methods are available to measure these values directly[2,4,10,11]; the issue of which of these methods is best remains controversial.

Regardless of the measurement method used, the authors should report the source of the ratings. In a decision analysis built for an individual patient, the most (and probably only) credible ratings are those measured directly from that patient. For analyses built to inform clinical policy, credible ratings could come from 3 sources. First, they may come from direct measurements from a large group of patients with the disorder in question and to whom results of the decision analysis could be applied. Second, ratings may come from other published studies of quality-of-life judgments by such patients, as was done in an analysis of strategies for chronic atrial fibrillation.[12] Third, they may come from ratings made by an equally large group of people representing the general public. Whoever provides the rating must understand the outcomes they are asked to rate; the more the raters know about the condition, the more credible are their utility ratings.

Do the Authors Indicate the Strength of Their Recommendations?

Multiple considerations should inform the strength or grade of recommendations: the quality of the evidence, the magnitude of the intervention effects in different studies, the magnitude of adverse effects, the burden to the patient and the health care system, the costs, and the relative value placed on different outcomes. Thus, recommendations may vary from those that rely on evidence from a systematic review of RCTs that show large treatment effects on patient-important outcomes with minimal adverse effects, inconvenience, and costs (yielding a strong recommendation) to those that rely on evidence from observational studies showing a small magnitude of treatment effect with appreciable adverse effects and costs (yielding a weak recommendation).

There are 2 ways that those developing recommendations can indicate their strength. One, most appropriate for practice guidelines, is to formally grade the strength of a recommendation. The other, most appropriate for decision analyses, is to vary the assumptions about the effect of the management options on the outcomes of interest. In this latter approach, a sensitivity analysis, investigators explore the extent to which various assumptions might affect the ultimate recommendation. We will discuss the 2 approaches in turn.

Grades of Recommendation

The Canadian Task Force on the Periodic Health Examination proposed the first formal taxonomy of "levels of evidence"[34-36] focusing on individual studies. There has since been a gradual evolution of rating systems, which has included a tremendous proliferation in their number and variety.[37] An international group of methodologists and guideline developers, a number of whom also participated in producing this book, have created a framework for rating quality of evidence and strength of recommendations[38,39] that is being widely adopted.[37]

The grades of recommendation, assessment, development, and evaluation (GRADE) system classifies recommendations in one of 2 levels, strong and weak, and quality of evidence into one of 4 categories, high, moderate, low, and very low. Evidence based on RCTs begins with a top rating on GRADE's 4-category quality of evidence classification (Table 15-3). GRADE takes into account, however, that not all RCTs are alike and that limitations of individual RCTs may compromise the quality of their evidence, as may other factors, including inconsistency of results, indirect evidence, and a high likelihood of reporting bias (Table 15-4). Evidence based on observational studies begins with a low-quality rating but may move up to moderate or high if the effect size is large enough, the evident biases all favor conventional rather than experimental therapy, or a dose-response gradient is evident (Table 15-4).

TABLE 15-3

Quality of Evidence and Its Definitions

Grade	Definition
High	Further research is unlikely to change our confidence in the estimate of effect.
Moderate	Further research is likely to have an important influence on our confidence in the estimate of effect and may change the estimate.
Low	Further research is very likely to have an important influence on our confidence in the estimate of effect and is likely to change the estimate.
Very low	Any estimate of effect is uncertain.

TABLE 15-4

Factors in Deciding on Confidence in Estimates of Benefits, Risks, Burden, and Costs

Factors that may decrease the quality of evidence

1. Poor quality of planning or implementation of the available studies, suggesting high likelihood of bias
2. Inconsistency of results
3. Indirectness of evidence
4. Imprecise estimates
5. Publication bias

Factors that may increase the quality of evidence

1. Large magnitude of effect
2. All plausible confounding would reduce a demonstrated effect
3. Dose-response gradient

The GRADE system offers a strong recommendation when an intervention's benefits clearly outweigh its risks and burden or clearly do not. On the other hand, when the tradeoff between benefits and downsides is less certain, either because of low-quality evidence or because high-quality evidence suggests benefits and downsides are closely balanced, weak recommendations become appropriate. Table 15-5 provides a structure for applying the results of the GRADE system of presenting recommendations.

Sensitivity Analysis

Decision analysts use the systematic exploration of the uncertainty in the data, known as *sensitivity analysis*, to see what effects varying estimates for downsides, benefits, and values have on expected clinical outcomes and, therefore, on the choice of clinical strategies. Sensitivity analysis asks the question, is the conclusion generated by the decision analysis affected by the uncertainties in the estimates of the likelihood or value of the outcomes? Estimates can be varied one at a time, termed "1-way" sensitivity analyses, or can

TABLE 15-5

GRADE Recommendations

Grade of Recommendation	Benefit vs Risk and Burdens
Strong recommendation, high-quality evidence	Benefits clearly outweigh risk and burdens, or vice versa
Strong recommendation, moderate-quality evidence	Benefits clearly outweigh risk and burdens, or vice versa
Strong recommendation, low- or very-low-quality evidence	Benefits clearly outweigh risk and burdens, or vice versa
Weak recommendation, high-quality evidence	Benefits closely balanced with risks and burden
Weak recommendation, moderate-quality evidence	Benefits closely balanced with risks and burden
Weak recommendation, low- or very-low-quality evidence	Uncertainty in the estimates of benefits, risks, and burden; benefits, risk, and burden may be closely balanced

Abbreviations: GRADE, grades of recommendation, assessment, development, and evaluation; RCT, randomized controlled trial.

Methodologic Quality of Supporting Evidence	Implications
RCTs without important limitations or overwhelming evidence from observational studies	Strong recommendation; can apply to most patients in most circumstances without reservation
RCTs with important limitations (inconsistent results; methodologic flaws; indirect, imprecise, or high likelihood of reporting bias) or exceptionally strong evidence from observational studies	
Observational studies or case series	Strong recommendation but may change when higher-quality evidence becomes available
RCTs without important limitations	Weak recommendation; best action may differ, depending on circumstances or patient or societal values
RCTs with important limitations (inconsistent results; methodologic flaws; indirect, imprecise, or high likelihood of reporting bias)	
Observational studies or case series	Very weak recommendations; other alternatives may be equally reasonable

be varied 2 or more at a time, known as "multiway" sensitivity analyses. For instance, investigators conducting a decision analysis of the administration of antibiotic agents for prevention of *Mycobacterium avium intracellulare* in patients with human immunodeficiency virus found that the cost-effectiveness of prophylaxis decreased if they assumed either a longer lifespan for patients or made a less sanguine estimate of the drugs' effectiveness.[40] If they simultaneously assumed a longer lifespan and decreased drug effectiveness (a 2-way sensitivity analysis), the cost-effectiveness decreased substantially. Clinicians should look for a table that lists which variables the analysts included in their sensitivity analyses, what range of values they used for each variable, and which variables, if any, altered the choice of strategies.

Ideally, decision analysts will subject all of their probability estimates to a sensitivity analysis. The range over which they will test should depend on the source of the data. If the estimates come from large, high-quality, randomized trials with narrow confidence limits, the range of estimates tested can be narrow. When methods are less valid or estimates of benefits and downsides less precise, sensitivity analyses testing a wide range of values become appropriate.

Decision analysts should also test utility values with sensitivity analyses, with the range of values again determined by the source of the data. If large numbers of patients or knowledgeable and representative members of the general public gave similar ratings to the outcome states, investigators can use a narrow range of utility values in the sensitivity analyses. If the ratings came from a small group of raters, or if the values for individuals varied widely, then investigators should use a wider range of utility values in the sensitivity analyses.

To the extent that the result of the decision analysis does not change with varying probability estimates and varying values, clinicians can consider the recommendation a strong one. When the final decision shifts with different plausible values of probabilities or values, the recommendation becomes much weaker.

We have suggested 4 criteria that affect the validity of a recommendation (Table 15-1). Table 15-6 presents a scheme for classify-

TABLE 15-6

A Hierarchy of Rigor in Making Treatment Recommendations

Level of Rigor	Systematic Summary of Evidence	Considers All Relevant Options and Outcomes	Explicit Statement of Values	Sample Methodologies
High	Yes	Yes	Yes	Practice guideline or decision analysis[a]
Intermediate	Yes	Yes or no	No	Systematic review[a]
Low	No	Yes or no	No	Traditional review; article reporting primary research

[a]Sample methodologies may not reflect the level of rigor shown. Exceptions may occur in either direction. For example, if the author of a practice guideline or decision analysis neither systematically collects nor summarizes information and if neither societal nor patient values are explicitly considered, recommendations will be produced that are of low rigor. Conversely, if the author of a systematic review does consider all relevant options and at least qualitatively considers values, the recommendations from the review may be rigorous.

ing the methodologic quality of treatment recommendations, emphasizing the 3 key components: consideration of all relevant options and outcomes, a systematic summary of the evidence, and an explicit or quantitative consideration, or both, of societal or patient preferences.

Are Treatment Recommendations Desirable at All?

The approaches we have described highlight the view that patient management decisions are always a function of both evidence and values and preferences. Values may differ substantially among settings. For example, monitoring of anticoagulant therapy might take on a much stronger negative value in a rural setting in which travel distances are large or in a more severely resource-constrained environment in which there is a direct inverse relationship between the resources available for purchase of antibiotic drugs and those allocated to monitoring levels of anticoagulation.

Patient-to-patient differences in values are equally important. The magnitude of the negative value of anticoagulant monitoring or the relative negative value associated with a stroke vs a gastrointestinal bleeding episode will vary widely among individual patients, even in the same setting.

If decisions are so dependent on preferences, what is the point of recommendations? Perhaps, rather than making recommendations, investigators should systematically search for, accumulate, and summarize information for presentation to clinicians. In addition, they may highlight the implications of different sets of values for clinical action. The dependence of any decision on patients' underlying values—and the variability of values—would suggest that such a presentation would be more useful than a recommendation.

Although this approach might be work in an ideal world, it is not well suited to the one in which we live. Its implementation depends on investigators using standard, rigorous methods of summarizing and presenting information and on clinicians having the time, energy, and skills to both interpret the summaries and integrate them with patient values and preferences. These requirements are unlikely to be met in the foreseeable future. Recommendations help clinicians practice efficiently, and applying the concepts of this chapter will allow clinicians to restrict their use of recommendations to those of high methodologic quality.

CLINICAL RESOLUTION

Returning to our opening clinical scenario,[26] you begin by considering whether the guideline developers have addressed all important patient groups, treatment options, and outcomes. You observe that they make separate recommendations for patients with various risk of stroke but not for patients with different risk of bleeding. The latter omission may occur because studies of prognosis have been inconsistent in the apparent risk factors for bleeding they identified. The guideline addresses the options you are seriously considering (full- and fixed-dose warfarin and aspirin) and major outcomes of interest (occlusive [embolic] stroke, hemorrhagic stroke, gastrointestinal bleeding, and other major bleeding events) but does not deal specifically with the need for regular blood testing or the frequent minor bruising and worries about bleeding associated with warfarin therapy.

Moving to the selection and synthesis of the evidence, you find the guideline's eligibility criteria to be appropriate and the supportive literature search to be comprehensive. The synthesis method, although not explicit, clearly relies on systematic reviews and meta-analyses.

The authors of the guideline make it clear that they believe patient values are crucial to the decision and do a good job of articulating the tradeoff.

> Underlying values and preferences: Anticoagulation with warfarin has far greater efficacy than aspirin in preventing stroke, and particularly in preventing severe ischemic stroke, in atrial fibrillation. We recommend the option of aspirin therapy for lower-risk groups, estimating that the absolute expected benefit of anticoagulant therapy may not be worth the increased hemorrhagic risk and burden of anticoagulation. Individual lower-risk patients may rationally choose anticoagulation over aspirin therapy to gain greater protection against ischemic stroke if they value protection against stroke much more highly than reducing risk of hemorrhage and burden of managing anticoagulation.

The guideline developers present approaches for determining stroke risk: for this patient, the risk is approximately 4%. They use a grading system that is a predecessor to the one presented earlier in this chapter (Table 15-5) and is similar. For patients such as those in the scenario, the guideline developers provide a strong recommendation, based on high-quality evidence, for use of warfarin. Given that the guideline meets all the criteria of Table 15-2, you are inclined to take this recommendation seriously.

The decision analysis that you identified[2] restricts its comparison to warfarin therapy vs no treatment. Its rationale for omitting aspirin is that its efficacy is not proven (although the aspirin effect in other meta-analyses has achieved statistical significance, it has always been borderline). The investigators do not mention any other antiplatelet treatment. They include outcomes of the inconvenience associated with monitoring of anticoagulant therapy, major bleeding episodes, mild stroke, severe stroke, and cost. They omit minor bleeding.

The investigators present their search strategies clearly. They restrict themselves to the results of computer searches of the published literature but, given this limitation, their searches appear comprehensive. With great clarity, they also describe their rationale for selecting evidence, and their criteria appear rigorous. They note the limitations of one key decision: to choose data from the Framingham study, rather than from RCTs of therapy for patients with atrial fibrillation, from which to derive their risk estimates.

To generate values, the authors interviewed 57 community-dwelling elderly people with a mean age of 73 years. They used standard gamble methodology to generate utility values. Their key values include utilities, on a 0 to 1.0 scale in which 0 is death and 1.0 is full health, of 0.986 for warfarin managed by a general practitioner, 0.880 for a major bleeding episode, 0.675 for a mild stroke, and 0 for a severe stroke.

The investigators conducted a sensitivity analysis that indicated their model was sensitive to variation in patients' utility for taking warfarin. If they assumed utility values for taking warfarin in the upper quartile (1.0; that is, no disutility is suggested for taking warfarin), their analysis suggests that virtually all patients should be receiving warfarin treatment. If they assumed the lower quartile utility (0.92), the analysis suggests that most patients should not be taking warfarin.

This decision analysis rates high with respect to the validity criteria in Table 15-2. The utilities in the investigators' core analysis using best estimates of risk and risk reduction (their *base case* analysis) match those of the patient in the scenario well. The investigators provided tables that suggest the best decision for different patients; when we add the characteristics of the patient being considered in the opening scenario, we find that this patient fits into a cell near the boundary between "no benefit" and "clear benefit," and the investigators' sensitivity analysis suggests that if she places the same value on life while taking warfarin than life while not taking warfarin, she would benefit from using the drug.

Having reviewed what turns out to be a rigorous guideline and a rigorous decision analysis, you are in a much stronger position to help the patient with her decision. It is clear to you that you need to explore her feelings about how she would tolerate the inconvenience and bleeding risk associated with taking warfarin. Your preference is for a shared decision-making style, and in preparation for the discussion with the patient, you note the high value you place on stroke prevention and your assessment that it would be in the patient's best interests to be taking warfarin.

References

1. Singer DE, Albers GW, Dalen JE, Go AS, Halperin JL, Manning WJ. Antithrombotic therapy in atrial fibrillation: the Seventh ACCP Conference on Antithrombotic and Thrombolytic Therapy. *Chest.* 2004;126(3)(suppl):429S-456S.

2. Thomson R, Parkin D, Eccles M, Sudlow M, Robinson A. Decision analysis and guidelines for anticoagulant therapy to prevent stroke in patients with atrial fibrillation. *Lancet.* 2000;355(9208):956-962.

3. Vandenbroucke-Grauls CM, Vandenbroucke JP. Effect of selective decontamination of the digestive tract on respiratory tract infections and mortality in the intensive care unit. *Lancet.* 1991;338(8771):859-862.

4. Selective Decontamination of the Digestive Tract Trialists' Collaborative Group. Meta-analysis of randomised controlled trials of selective decontamination of the digestive tract. *BMJ.* 1993;307(6903):525-532.

5. Heyland DK, Cook DJ, Jaeschke R, Griffith L, Lee HN, Guyatt GH. Selective decontamination of the digestive tract: an overview. *Chest.* 1994;105(4): 1221-1229.

6. Kollef MH. The role of selective digestive tract decontamination on mortality and respiratory tract infections: a meta-analysis. *Chest.* 1994; 105(4):1101-1108.

7. Glasziou PP, Irwig LM. An evidence based approach to individualising treatment. *BMJ.* 1995;311(7016):1356-1359.

8. Sinclair JC, Cook RJ, Guyatt GH, Pauker SG, Cook DJ. When should an effective treatment be used? derivation of the threshold number needed to treat and the minimum event rate for treatment. *J Clin Epidemiol.* 2006;54(3):217-324.

9. Smith GD, Egger M. Who benefits from medical interventions? *BMJ.* 1994;308(6921):72-74.

10. Field MJ, Lohr KN, eds. *Clinical Practice Guidelines. Directions for a New Program.* Washington, DC: National Academy Press; 1990.

11. American Medical Association Specialty *Society Practice Parameters Partnership and Practice Parameters Forum. Attributes to Guide the Development of Practice Parameters.* Chicago, IL: American Medical Association; 1990.

12. American College of Physicians. *Clinical Efficacy Assessment Project: Procedural Manual.* Philadelphia, PA: American College of Physicians; 1986.

13. Gottlieb LK, Margolis CZ, Schoenbaum SC. Clinical practice guidelines at an HMO: development and implementation in a quality improvement model. *QRB Qual Rev Bull.* 1990;16(2):80-86.

14. Lohr KN, Field MJ. A provisional instrument for assessing clinical practice guidelines. In: Field MJ, Lohr KN, eds. *Guidelines for Clinical Practice: From Development to Use.* Washington, DC: National Academy Press; 1992:346-410.

15. Harris RP, Helfand M, Woolf SH, et al; Methods Work Group, Third US Preventive Services Task Force. Current Methods of the US Preventive Services Task Force: a review of the process. *Am J Prev Med*. 2001;20(3 suppl):21-35.

16. Park RE, Fink A, Brook RH, et al. Physician ratings of appropriate indications for six medical and surgical procedures. *Am J Public Health*. 1986;76(7):766-772.

17. Keeney RL. Decision analysis: an overview. *Oper Res*. 1982;30(5):803-838.

18. Eckman MH, Levine HJ, Pauker SG. Decision analytic and cost-effectiveness issues concerning anticoagulant prophylaxis in heart disease. *Chest*. 1992;102(4)(suppl):538S-549S.

19. Kassirer JP, Moskowitz AJ, Lau J, Pauker SG. Decision analysis: a progress report. *Ann Intern Med*. 1987;106(2):275-291.

20. Eddy DM. Clinical decision making: from theory to practice: designing a practice policy: standards, guidelines, and options. *JAMA*. 1990;263(22): 3077, 3081, 3084.

21. Drummond MF, Richardson WS, O'Brien BJ, Levine M, Heyland D. Users' guides to the medical literature, XIII: how to use an article on economic analysis of clinical practice, A: are the results of the study valid? Evidence Based Medicine Working Group. *JAMA*. 1997;277(19):1552-1557.

22. O'Brien BJ, Heyland D, Richardson WS, Levine M, Drummond MF. Users' guides to the medical literature, XIII: how to use an article on economic analysis of clinical practice, B: what are the results and will they help me in caring for my patients? Evidence-Based Medicine Working Group. *JAMA*. 1997;277(22):1802-1806.

23. Matchar DB, McCrory DC, Barnett HJ, Feussner JR. Medical treatment for stroke prevention. *Ann Intern Med*. 1994;121(1):41-53.

24. American College of Physicians. Guidelines for medical treatment for stroke prevention. *Ann Intern Med*. 1994;121(1):54-55.

25. North American Symptomatic Carotid Endarterectomy Trial Collaborators. Beneficial effect of carotid endarterectomy in symptomatic patients with high-grade carotid stenosis. *N Engl J Med*. 1991;325(7):445-453.

26. Jackson R, Lawes CM, Bennett DA, Milne RJ, Rodgers A. Treatment with drugs to lower blood pressure and blood cholesterol based on an individual's absolute cardiovascular risk. *Lancet*. 2005;365(9457):434-441.

27. Tsevat J, Eckman MH, McNutt RA, Pauker SG. Warfarin for dilated cardiomyopathy: a bloody tough pill to swallow? *Med Decis Making*. 1989;9(3):162-169.

28. Taylor R, Giles J. Cash interests taint drug advice. *Nature*. 2005;43 7(7062):1070-1071.

29. Laupacis A. On bias and transparency in the development of influential recommendations. *CMAJ*. 2006;174(3):335-336.

30. *CMAJ*. Clinical practice guidelines and conflict of interest. *CMAJ.* 2005;173(11): 1297, 1299.

31. CAPRIE Steering Committee. A randomised, blinded, trial of clopidogrel versus aspirin in patients at risk of ischaemic events (CAPRIE). *Lancet.* 1996;348(9038):1329-1339.

32. Albers GW, Amarenco P, Easton JD, Sacco RL, Teal P. Antithrombotic and thrombolytic therapy for ischemic stroke: the Seventh ACCP Conference on Antithrombotic and Thrombolytic Therapy. *Chest.* 2004;126(3)(suppl):483S-512S.

33. Clagett GP, Sobel M, Jackson MR, Lip GY, Tangelder M, Verhaeghe R. Antithrombotic therapy in peripheral arterial occlusive disease: the Seventh ACCP Conference on Antithrombotic and Thrombolytic Therapy. *Chest.* 2004;126(3)(suppl):609S-626S.

34. Canadian Task Force on the Periodic Health Examination. The periodic health examination. *CMAJ.* 1979;121(9):1193-1254.

35. Woolf SH, Battista RN, Anderson GM, Logan AG, Wang E. Assessing the clinical effectiveness of preventive maneuvers: analytic principles and systematic methods in reviewing evidence and developing clinical practice recommendations: a report by the Canadian Task Force on the Periodic Health Examination. *J Clin Epidemiol.* 1990;43(9):891-905.

36. Sackett DL. Rules of evidence and clinical recommendations on the use of antithrombotic agents. *Chest.* 1986;89(2 suppl):2S-4S.

37. Guyatt G, Vist G, Falck-Ytter Y, Kunz R, Magrini N, Schunemann H. An emerging consensus on grading recommendations? *ACP J Club.* 2006; 144(1):A8-A9.

38. Atkins D, Best D, Briss PA, et al. Grading quality of evidence and strength of recommendations. *BMJ.* 2004;328(7454):1490.

39. Guyatt G, Gutterman D, Baumann MH, et al. Grading strength of recommendations and quality of evidence in clinical guidelines: report from an American College of Chest Physicians task force. *Chest.* 2006;129(1):174-181.

40. Bayoumi AM, Redelmeier DA. Preventing *Mycobacterium avium* complex in patients who are using protease inhibitors: a cost-effectiveness analysis. *AIDS.* 1998;12(12):1503-1512.

GLOSSARY

Term	Definition
Absolute Difference	The absolute difference in rates of good or harmful outcomes between experimental groups (experimental event rate, or EER) and control groups (control event rate, or CER), calculated as the event rate in the experimental group minus the event rate in the control group (EER – CER). For instance, if the rate of adverse events is 20% in the control group and 10% in the treatment group, the absolute difference is 20% – 10% = 10%.
Absolute Risk (or Baseline Risk or Control Event Rate [CER])	The risk of an event (eg, if 10 of 100 patients have an event, the absolute risk is 10% expressed as a percentage, or 0.10 expressed as a proportion).
Absolute Risk Increase (ARI)	The absolute difference in rates of harmful outcomes between experimental groups (experimental event rate, or EER) and control groups (control event rate, or CER), calculated as rate of harmful outcome in experimental group minus rate of harmful outcome in control group (EER – CER). Typically used to describe a harmful exposure or intervention (eg, if the rate of adverse outcomes is 20% in treatment and 10% in control, the absolute risk increase would be 10% expressed as a percentage and 0.10 expressed as a proportion).
Absolute Risk Reduction (ARR) or Risk Difference	The absolute difference (risk difference) in rates of harmful outcomes between experimental groups (experimental event rate, or EER) and control groups (control event rate, or CER), calculated as the rate of harmful outcome in the control group minus the rate of harmful outcome in the experimental group (CER – EER). Typically used to describe a beneficial exposure or intervention (eg, if 20% of patients in the control group have an adverse event, as do 10% among treated patients, the ARR or risk difference would be 10% expressed as a percentage or 0.10 expressed as a proportion).

Term	Definition
Academic Detailing (or Educational Outreach Visits)	A strategy for changing clinician behavior. Use of a trained person who meets with professionals in their practice settings to provide information with the intent of changing their practice. The pharmaceutical industry frequently uses this strategy, to which the term *detailing* is applied. Academic detailing is such an interaction initiated by an academic group or institution rather than the pharmaceutical industry.
Adherence (or Compliance)	Extent to which patients carry out health care recommendations, or the extent to which health care providers carry out the diagnostic tests, monitoring equipment, interventional requirements, and other technical specifications that define optimal patient management.
Adjusted Analysis	An adjusted analysis takes into account differences in prognostic factors (or baseline characteristics) between groups that may influence the outcome. For instance, when comparing an experimental and control intervention, if the experimental group is on average older, and thus at higher risk of an adverse outcome than the control group, the analysis adjusted for age will show a larger treatment effect than the unadjusted analysis.
Alerting (or Alerting Systems)	A strategy for changing clinician behavior. A type of computer decision support system that alerts the clinician to a circumstance that might require clinical action (eg, a system that highlights out-of-range laboratory values).
Algorithm	An explicit description of an ordered sequence of steps with branching logic that can be applied under specific clinical circumstances. The logic of an algorithm is: if *a*, then do *x*; if *b*, then do *y*; etc.
Allocation Concealment (or Concealment)	Randomization is concealed if the person who is making the decision about enrolling a patient is unaware of whether the next patient enrolled will be entered in the intervention or control group (using techniques such as central randomization or sequentially numbered opaque sealed envelopes). If randomization is not concealed, patients with differing prognosis may be differentially recruited to treatment or control groups. Of particular concern, patients with better prognoses may tend to be preferentially enrolled in the active treatment arm, resulting in exaggeration of the apparent benefit of the intervention (or even the false conclusion that the intervention is efficacious).

Term	Definition
α Level	The probability of erroneously concluding there is a difference between comparison groups when there is in fact no difference (type I error). Typically, investigators decide on the chance of a false-positive result they are willing to accept when they plan the sample size for a study (eg, investigators often set α level at .05).
Audit and Feedback	A strategy for changing clinician behavior. Any written or verbal summary of clinician performance (eg, based on chart review or observation of clinical practice) during a period of time. The summary may also include recommendations to improve practice.
Background Questions	These clinical questions are about physiology, pathology, epidemiology, and general management and are often asked by clinicians in training. The answers to background questions are often best found in textbooks or narrative review articles
Base Case	In an economic evaluation, the base case is the best estimates of each of the key variables that bear on the costs and effects of the alternative management strategies.
Baseline Characteristics	Factors that describe study participants at the beginning of the study (eg, age, sex, disease severity); in comparison studies, it is important that these characteristics be initially similar between groups; if not balanced or if the imbalance is not statistically adjusted, these characteristics can cause confounding and can bias study results.
Baseline Risk (or Baseline Event Rate or Control Event Rate [CER])	The proportion or percentage of study participants in the control group in whom an adverse outcome is observed.
Bayesian Diagnostic Reasoning	The essence of bayesian reasoning is that one starts with a prior probability or probability distribution and incorporates new information to arrive at a posterior probability or probability distribution. The approach to diagnosis presented in this book assumes that diagnosticians are intuitive bayesian thinkers and move from pretest to posttest probabilities as information accumulates.
Before-After Design (or One-Group Pretest-Posttest Design)	Study in which the investigators compare the status of a group of study participants before and after the implementation of an intervention.

Term	Definition
Bias (or Systematic Error)	Systematic deviation from the underlying truth because of a feature of the design or conduct of a research study (for example, overestimation of a treatment effect because of failure to randomize). Sometimes, authors label specific types of bias in a variety of contexts.

1. Channeling Effect or Channeling Bias: Tendency of clinicians to prescribe treatment according to a patient's prognosis. As a result of the behavior, in observational studies, treated patients are more or less likely to be high-risk patients than untreated patients, leading to biased estimate of treatment effect.

2. Data Completeness Bias: Using a computer decision support system (CDSS) to log episodes in the intervention group and using a manual system in the non-CDSS control group can create variation in the completeness of data.

3. Detection Bias (or Surveillance Bias): Tendency to look more carefully for an outcome in one of the comparison groups.

4. Differential Verification Bias: When test results influence the choice of the reference standard (eg, test-positive patients undergo an invasive test to establish the diagnosis, whereas test-negative patients undergo long-term follow-up without application of the invasive test) the assessment of test properties may be biased.

5. Expectation Bias: In data collection, an interviewer has information that influences his or her expectation of finding the exposure or outcome. In clinical practice, a clinician's assessment may be influenced by previous knowledge of the presence or absence of a disorder.

6. Incorporation Bias: Occurs when investigators use a reference standard that incorporates a diagnostic test that is the subject of investigation. The result is a bias toward making the test appear more powerful in differentiating target positive from target negative than it actually is.

(Continued)

Term	Definition
Bias (or Systematic Error) (*Continued*)	7. Interviewer Bias: Greater probing by an interviewer of some participants than others, contingent on particular features of the participants.
	8. Lead Time Bias: Occurs when outcomes such as survival, as measured from the time of diagnosis, may be increased not because patients live longer, but because screening lengthens the time that they know they have disease.
	9. Length Time Bias: Occurs when patients whose disease is discovered by screening also may appear to do better or live longer than people whose disease presents clinically with symptoms because screening tends to detect disease that is destined to progress slowly and that therefore has a good prognosis.
	10. Observer Bias: Occurs when an observer's observations differ systematically according to participant characteristics (eg, making systematically different observations in treatment and control groups).
	11. Partial Verification Bias: Occurs when only a selected sample of patients who underwent the index test is verified by the reference standard, and that sample is dependent on the results of the test. For example, patients with suspected coronary artery disease whose exercise test results are positive may be more likely to undergo coronary angiography (the reference standard) than those whose exercise test results are negative.
	12. Publication Bias: Occurs when the publication of research depends on the direction of the study results and whether they are statistically significant.
	13. Recall Bias: Occurs when patients who experience an adverse outcome have a different likelihood of recalling an exposure than patients who do not experience the adverse outcome, independent of the true extent of exposure.

(Continued)

Term	Definition
Bias (or Systematic Error) (*Continued*)	14. Referral Bias: Occurs when characteristics of patients differ between one setting (such as primary care) and another setting that includes only referred patients (such as secondary or tertiary care).
	15. Reporting Bias (or selective outcome reporting bias): The inclination of authors to differentially report research results according toto the magnitude, direction, or statistical significance of the results.
	16. Social Desirability Bias: Occurs when participants answer according to social norms or socially desirable behavior rather than what is actually the case (for instance, underreporting alcohol consumption).
	17. Spectrum Bias: Ideally, diagnostic test properties will be assessed in a population in which the spectrum of disease in the target-positive patients includes all those in whom clinicians might be uncertain about the diagnosis, and the target-negative patients include all those with conditions easily confused with the target condition. Spectrum bias may occur when the accuracy of a diagnostic test is assessed in a population that differs from this ideal. Examples of spectrum bias would include a situation in which a substantial proportion of the target-positive population have advanced disease and target-negative participants are normal or asymptomatic. Such situations typically occur in diagnostic case-control studies (for instance, comparing those with advanced disease to normal individuals). Such studies are liable to yield an overly sanguine estimate of the usefulness of the test.
	18. Surveillance Bias. See Detection Bias.
	19. Verification Bias. See Differential Verification bias.
	20. Workup Bias. See Differential Verification Bias.
Binary Outcome	See Dichotomous outcome.

Term	Definition
Blind (or Blinded or Masked)	Patients, clinicians, data collectors, outcome adjudicators, or data analysts unaware of which patients have been assigned to the experimental or control group. In the case of diagnostic tests, those interpreting the test results are unaware of the result of the reference standard or vice versa.
Boolean Operators (or Logical Operators)	Words used when searching electronic databases. These operators are AND, OR, and NOT and are used to combine terms (AND/OR) or exclude terms (NOT) from the search strategy.
Bootstrap Technique	A statistical technique for estimating parameters such as standard errors and confidence intervals based on resampling from an observed data set with replacement from the original sample.
Case-Control Study	A study designed to determine the association between an exposure and outcome in which patients are sampled by outcome. Those with the outcome (cases) are compared with those without the outcome (controls) with respect to exposure to the suspected harmful agent.
Case Series	A report of a study of a collection of patients treated in a similar manner, without a control group. For example, a clinician might describe the characteristics of an outcome for 25 consecutive patients with diabetes who received education for prevention of foot ulcers.
Case Study	In qualitative research, an exploration of a case defined by some boundaries or contemporary phenomena usually within a real-life context.
Categorical Variable	A categorical variable may be nominal or ordinal. Categorical variables can be defined according to attributes without any associated order (eg, medical admission, elective surgery, or emergency surgery); these are called nominal variables. A categorical variable can also be defined according to attributes that are ordered (eg, height such as high, medium, or low); these are called ordinal variables.
Chance-Corrected Agreement	The proportion of possible agreement achieved beyond that which one would expect by chance alone, often measured by the φ statistic.

Term	Definition
Chance-Independent Agreement	The proportion of possible agreement achieved that is independent of chance and unaffected by the distribution of ratings, as measured by the φ statistic.
Channeling Effect or Channeling Bias	See Bias.
Checklist Effect	The improvement seen in medical decision making because of more complete and structured data collection (eg, clinicians fill out a detailed form, so their decisions improve).
χ^2 Test	A nonparametric test of statistical significance used to compare the distribution of categorical outcomes in 2 or more groups, the null hypothesis of which is that the underlying distributions are identical.
Class Effect (or Drug Class Effect)	When similar effects are produced by most or all members of a class of drugs (eg, β-blockers or calcium antagonists).
Clinical Decision Rules (or Decision Rules, Clinical Prediction Rules, or Prediction Rules)	A guide for practice that is generated by initially examining, and ultimately combining, a number of variables to predict the likelihood of a current diagnosis or a future event. Sometimes, if the likelihood is sufficiently high or low, the rule generates a suggested course of action.
Clinical Decision Support System	A strategy for changing clinician behavior. An information system used to integrate clinical and patient information and provide support for decision-making in patient care. See also Computer Decision Support System.
Clinical Practice Guidelines (or Guidelines or Practice Guidelines)	A strategy for changing clinician behavior. Systematically developed statements or recommendations to assist practitioner and patient decisions about appropriate health care for specific clinical circumstances.
Cluster Analysis	A statistical procedure in which the unit of analysis matches the unit of randomization, which is something other than the patient or participant (eg, school, clinic).

Term	Definition
Cluster Assignment (or Cluster Randomization)	The assignment of groups (eg, schools, clinics) rather than individuals to intervention and control groups. This approach is often used when assignment by individuals is likely to result in contamination (eg, if adolescents within a school are assigned to receive or not receive a new sex education program, it is likely that they will share the information they learn with one another; instead, if the unit of assignment is schools, entire schools are assigned to receive or not receive the new sex education program). Cluster assignment is typically randomized, but it is possible (though not advisable) to assign clusters to treatment or control by other methods.
Cochrane Q	A common test for heterogeneity that assumes the null hypothesis that all the apparent variability between individual study results is due to chance. Cochrane Q generates a probability, presented as a P value, based on a χ^2 distribution, that between-study differences in results equal to or greater than those observed are likely to occur simply by chance.
Cohort	A group of persons with a common characteristic or set of characteristics. Typically, the group is followed for a specified period to determine the incidence of a disorder or complications of an established disorder (prognosis).
Cohort Study (or Longitudinal Study or Prospective Study)	This is an investigation in which a cohort of individuals who do not have evidence of an outcome of interest but who are exposed to the putative cause is compared with a concurrent cohort of individuals who are also free of the outcome but not exposed to the putative cause. Both cohorts are then followed forward in time to compare the incidence of the outcome of interest. When used to study the effectiveness of an intervention, it is an investigation in which a cohort of individuals who receive the intervention is compared with a concurrent cohort who does not receive the intervention, wherein both cohorts are followed forward to compare the incidence of the outcome of interest. Cohort studies can be conducted retrospectively in the sense that someone other than the investigator has followed patients, and the investigator obtains the data base and then examines the association between exposure and outcome.

Term	Definition
Cointerventions	Interventions other than intervention under study that affect the outcome of interest and that may be differentially applied to intervention and control groups and thus potentially bias the result of a study.
Comorbidity	Disease(s) or conditions that coexist in study participants in addition to the index condition that is the subject of the study.
Compliance (or Adherence)	See Adherence.
Composite Endpoint (or Composite Outcome)	When investigators measure the effect of treatment on an aggregate of endpoints of various importance, this is a composite endpoint. Inferences from composite endpoints are strongest in the rare situations in which (1) the component endpoints are of similar patient importance, (2) the endpoints that are more important occur with at least similar frequency to those that are less important, and (3) strong biologic rationale supports results that, across component endpoints, show similar relative risks with sufficiently narrow confidence intervals.
Computer Decision Support System (CDSS)	A strategy for changing clinician behavior. Computer-based information systems used to integrate clinical and patient information and provide support for decision making in patient care. In clinical decision support systems that are computer based, detailed individual patient data are entered into a computer program and are sorted and matched to programs or algorithms in a computerized database, resulting in the generation of patient-specific assessments or recommendations. CDSSs can have the following purposes: alerting, reminding, critiquing, interpreting, predicting, diagnosing, and suggesting. See also Clinical Decision Support System.
Concealment (or Allocation Concealment)	See Allocation Concealment.
Concepts	The basic building blocks of theory.

Term	Definition
Conceptual Framework	An organization of interrelated ideas or concepts that provides a system of relationships between those ideas or concepts.
Conditional Probabilities	The probability of a particular state, given another state (ie, the probability of A, given B).
Confidence Interval (CI)	Range of values within which it is probable that the true value of a parameter (eg, a mean, a relative risk) lies.
Conflict of Interest	A conflict of interest exists when investigators, authors, institutions, reviewers, or editors have financial or nonfinancial relationships with other persons or organizations (such as study sponsors), or personal investments in research projects or the outcomes of projects, that may inappropriately influence their interpretation or actions. Conflicts of interest can lead to biased design, conduct, analysis, and interpretation of study results
Confounder (or Confounding Variable or Confounding)	A factor that is associated with the outcome of interest and is differentially distributed in patients exposed and unexposed to the outcome of interest.
Consecutive Sample (or Sequential Sample)	A sample in which all potentially eligible patients treated throughout a period are enrolled.
Consequentialist (or Utilitarian)	A consequentialist or utilitarian view of distributive justice contends that, even in individual decision making, the clinician should take a broad social view, favoring actions that provide the greatest good to the greatest number. In this broader view, the effect on others of allocating resources to a particular patient's care would bear on the decision. This is an alternative to the deontologic view.
Construct Validity	In measurement theory, a construct is a theoretically derived notion of the domain(s) we wish to measure. An understanding of the construct will lead to expectations about how an instrument should behave if it is valid. Construct validity therefore involves comparisons between the instrument being evaluated and other measures (eg, characteristics of patients or other scores) and the logical relationships that should exist between them.

Term	Definition
Contamination	Occurs when participants in either the experimental or control group receive the intervention intended for the other arm of the study.
Continuous Variable (or Interval Data)	A variable that can theoretically take any value and in practice can take a large number of values with small differences between them (eg, height). Continuous variables are also sometimes called interval data.
Control Event Rate (CER) (or Baseline Risk or Baseline Event Rate)	See Baseline Risk.
Control Group	A group that does not receive the experimental intervention. In many studies, the control group receives either usual care or a placebo.
Controlled Time Series Design (or Controlled Interrupted Time Series)	Data are collected at several times both before and after the intervention in the intervention group and at the same times in a control group. Data collected before the intervention allow the underlying trend and cyclical (seasonal) effects to be estimated. Data collected after the intervention allow the intervention effect to be estimated while accounting for underlying secular trends. Use of a control group addresses the greatest threat to the validity of a time series design, which is the occurrence of another event at the same time as the intervention, both of which may be associated with the outcome.
Correlation	The magnitude of the relationship between 2 variables.
Correlation Coefficient	A numeric expression of the magnitude and direction of the relationship between 2 variables, which can take values from –1.0 (perfect negative relationship) to 0 (no relationship) to 1.0 (perfect positive relationship).
Cost Analysis	An economic analysis in which only costs of various alternatives are compared. This comparison informs only the resource-use half of the decision (the other half being the expected outcomes).
Cost-Benefit Analysis	An economic analysis in which both the costs and the consequences (including increases in the length and quality of life) are expressed in monetary terms.

Term	Definition
Cost-Effectiveness Acceptability Curve	The cost-effectiveness acceptability is plotted on a graph that relates the maximum one is willing to pay for a particular treatment alternative (eg, how many dollars one is willing to pay to gain 1 life-year) on the x-axis to the probability that a treatment alternative is cost-effective compared with all other treatment alternatives on the y-axis. The curves are generated from uncertainty around the point estimates of costs and effects in trial-based economic evaluations or uncertainty around values for variables used in decision analytic models. As one is willing to pay more for health outcomes, treatment alternatives that initially might be considered unattractive (eg, a high cost per life-year saved) will have a higher probability of becoming more cost-effective. Cost-effectiveness acceptability curves are a convenient method of presenting the effect of uncertainty on economic evaluation results on a single figure instead of through the use of numerous tables and figures of sensitivity analyses.
Cost-Effectiveness Analysis	An economic analysis in which the consequences are expressed in natural units (eg, cost per life saved or cost per bleeding event averted). Sometimes, cost-utility analysis is classified as a subcategory of cost-effectiveness analysis.
Cost-Effectiveness Efficiency Frontier	The cost and effectiveness results of each treatment alternative from an economic evaluation can be graphed on a figure known as the cost-effectiveness plane. The cost-effectiveness plane plots cost on the vertical axis (ie, positive infinity at the top and negative infinity and the bottom) and effects such as life-years on the horizontal axis (ie, negative infinity at the far left and positive infinity at the far right). One treatment alternative such as usual care is plotted at the origin (ie, 0, 0) and all other treatment alternatives are plotted relative to the treatment at the origin. Treatment alternatives are considered dominated if they have both higher costs and lower effectiveness relative to any other. Line segments can be drawn connecting the nondominated treatment alternatives and the combination of line segments that join these nondominated treatment alternatives is referred to as the cost-effectiveness efficiency frontier. Constructed in this way, any treatment alternative that lies above the cost-effectiveness efficiency frontier is considered to be inefficient (dominated) by a treatment alternative or combination of alternatives on the efficiency frontier.

Term	Definition
Cost-Minimization Analysis	An economic analysis conducted in situations in which the consequences of the alternatives are identical and the only issue is their relative costs.
Cost-to-Charge Ratio	Where there is a systematic deviation between costs and charges, an economic analysis may adjust charges using a cost-to-charge ratio to approximate real costs.
Cost-Utility Analysis	A type of economic analysis in which the consequences are expressed in terms of life-years adjusted by peoples' preferences. Typically, one considers the incremental cost per incremental gain in quality-adjusted life-years (QALYs).
Cox Regression Model	A regression technique that allows adjustment for known differences in baseline characteristics or time-dependent characteristics between 2 groups applied to survival data.
Credibility (or Trustworthiness)	In qualitative research, a term used instead of validity to reflect whether the investigators engaged thoroughly and sensitively with the material and whether the investigators' interpretations are credible. Signs of credibility can be found not only in the procedural descriptions of methodology but also through an assessment of the coherence and depth of the findings reported.
Criterion Standard (or Gold Standard or Reference Standard)	A method having established or widely accepted accuracy for determining a diagnosis that provides a standard to which a new screening or diagnostic test can be compared. The method need not be a single or simple procedure but could include patient follow-up to observe the evolution of their condition or the consensus of an adjudication committee about their outcome.
Critical Theory	A qualitative research tradition focused on understanding the nature of power relationships and related constructs, often with the intention of helping to remedy systemic injustices in society.

Term	Definition
Critiquing (or Critiquing System)	A strategy for changing clinician behavior. A decision support approach in which the computer evaluates a clinician's decision and generates an appropriateness rating or an alternative suggestion.
Cronbach α Coefficient	Cronbach α is an index of reliability, homogeneity, or internal consistency of items on a measurement instrument. The Cronbach α increases with the magnitude of the interitem correlation and with the number of items.
Cross-Sectional Study	The observation of a defined population at a single point in time or during a specific interval. Exposure and outcome are determined simultaneously.
Data Completeness Bias	See Bias.
Data-Dredging	Searching a data set for differences between groups on particular outcomes, or in subgroups of patients, without explicit a priori hypotheses.
Decision Aid	A tool that endeavors to present patients with the benefits and harms of alternative courses of action in a manner that is quantitative, comprehensive, and understandable.
Decision Analysis	A systematic approach to decision making under conditions of uncertainty. It involves identifying all available alternatives and estimating the probabilities of potential outcomes associated with each alternative, valuing each outcome, and, on the basis of the probabilities and values, arriving at a quantitative estimate of the relative merit of each alternative.
Decision Rules (or Clinical Decision Rules)	See Clinical Decision Rules.
Decision Tree	Most clinical decision analyses are built as decision trees; articles usually will include 1 or more diagrams showing the structure of the decision tree used for the analysis.

Term	Definition
Degrees of Freedom	A technical term in a statistical analysis that has to do with the power of the analysis. The more degrees of freedom, the more powerful the analysis. The degrees of freedom typically refers to the number of observations in a sample minus the number of unknown parameters estimated for the model. It reflects a sort of adjusted sample size, with the adjustment based on the number of unknowns that need to be estimated in a model. For example, in a 2-sample t test the degrees of freedom is $n1 + n2 - 1 - 1$, because there are $n1 + n2$ subjects altogether and 1 mean estimated in one group and 1 mean in another, giving $n1 + n2 - 2$.
Deontologic	A deontologic approach to distributive justice holds that the clinician's only responsibility should be to best meet the needs of the individual under his or her care. This is an alternative to the consequentialist or utilitarian view.
Dependent Variable (or Outcome Variable or Target Variable)	The target variable of interest. The variable that is hypothesized to depend on or be caused by another variable, the independent variable.
Detection Bias (or Surveillance Bias)	See Bias.
Determinants of Outcome	The factors most strongly determining whether or not a target event will occur.
Dichotomous Outcome (or Binary Outcome)	A categorical variable that can take one of 2 discrete values rather than an incremental value on a continuum (eg, pregnant or not pregnant, dead or alive).
Differential Diagnosis (or Active Alternatives)	The set of diagnoses that can plausibly explain a patient's presentation.

Term	Definition
Differential Verification Bias	See Bias.
Directness	A key element to consider when grading the quality of evidence for a health care recommendation. Evidence is direct to the extent that study participants, interventions, and outcome measures are similar to those of interest.
Direct Observation	See Field Observation.
Discriminant Analysis	A statistical technique similar to logistic regression analysis that identifies variables that are associated with the presence or absence of a particular categorical (nominal) outcome.
Disease-Specific Health-Related Quality of Life	See Health-Related Quality of Life.
Document Analysis	In qualitative research, this is one of 3 basic data collection methods. It involves the interpretive review of written material.
Dominate	In economic evaluation, if the intervention of interest is both more effective and less costly than the control strategy, it is said to dominate the alternative.
Dose-Response Gradient (or Dose Dependence)	Exists when the risk of an outcome changes in the anticipated direction as the quantity or the duration of exposure to the putative harmful or beneficial agent increases.
Downstream Costs	Costs due to resources consumed in the future and associated with clinical events in the future that are attributable to the intervention.
Drug Class Effects (or Class Effects)	See Class Effects.

Term	Definition
Ecologic Study	Ecologic studies examine relationships between groups of individuals with exposure to a putative risk factor and an outcome. Exposures are measured at the population, community, or group level rather than at the individual level. Ecologic studies can provide information about an association; however, they are prone to bias: the ecologic fallacy. The ecologic fallacy holds that relationships observed for groups necessarily hold for individuals (eg, if countries with more dietary fat have higher rates of breast cancer, then women who eat fatty foods must be more likely to get breast cancer). These inferences may be correct but are only weakly supported by the aggregate data.
Economic Analysis (or Economic Evaluation)	A set of formal, quantitative methods used to compare 2 or more treatments, programs, or strategies with respect to their resource use and their expected outcomes.
Educational Meetings (or Interactive Workshops)	A strategy for changing clinician behavior. Participation of professionals in workshops that include interaction and discussion.
Educational Outreach Visits (or Academic Detailing)	See Academic Detailing.
Effect Size	The difference in outcomes between the intervention and control groups divided by some measure of variability, typically the standard deviation.
Efficiency	Technical efficiency is the relationship between inputs (costs) and outputs (in health, quality-adjusted life-years [QALYs]). Interventions that provide more QALYs for the same or fewer resources are more efficient. Technical efficiency is assessed using cost minimization, cost-effectiveness, and cost-utility analysis. Allocative efficiency recognizes that health is not the only goal that society wishes to pursue, so competing goals must be weighted and then related to costs. This is typically done through cost-benefit analysis.

Term	Definition
Efficiency Frontier	When the cost and effectiveness results of an economic evaluation are graphed on a cost-effectiveness plane along with incremental cost-effectiveness ratios, the resultant line segments are referred to as the efficiency frontier. Any strategy that has a base-case cost-effectiveness that is above the efficiency frontier would be considered dominated.
Endpoint	Event or outcome that leads to completion or termination of follow-up of an individual in a study (eg, death or major morbidity).
Equivalence Studies (or Equivalence Trial or Noninferiority Trials)	Trials that estimate treatment effects that exclude any patient-important superiority of interventions under evaluation are equivalence trials. Equivalence trials require a priori definition of the smallest difference in outcomes between these interventions that patients would consider large enough to justify a preference for the superior intervention (given the intervention's harms and burdens). The confidence interval for the estimated treatment effect at the end of the trial should exclude that difference for the authors to claim equivalence (ie, the confidence limits should be closer to zero than the minimal patient-important difference). This level of precision often requires investigators to enroll large number of patients with large number of events. Equivalence trials are helpful when investigators want to see whether a cheaper, safer, simpler (or increasingly often, better method to generate income for the sponsor) intervention is neither better nor worse (in terms of efficacy) than a current intervention. Claims of equivalence are frequent when results are not significant, but one must be alert to whether the confidence intervals exclude differences between the interventions that are as large as or larger than those patients would consider important. If they do not, the trial is indeterminate rather than yielding equivalence.
Ethnography (or Ethnographic Study)	In qualitative research, an approach to inquiry that focuses on the culture or subculture of a group of people to try to understand the world view of those under study.

Term	Definition
Event Rate	Proportion or percentage of study participants in a group in which an event is observed. Control event rate (CER) and experimental event rate (EER) are used to refer to event rates in control groups and experimental groups of study participants, respectively.
Evidence	A broad definition of evidence is any empirical observation, whether systematically collected or not. The unsystematic observations of the individual clinician constitute one source of evidence. Physiologic experiments constitute another source. Clinical research evidence refers to systematic observation of clinical events and is the focus of this book.
Evidence-Based Experts	Clinicians who can, in a sophisticated manner, independently find, appraise, and judiciously apply the best evidence to patient care.
Evidence-Based Health Care (EBHC)	The conscientious, explicit, and judicious use of current best evidence in making decisions about the care of individual patients. Evidence-based clinical practice requires integration of individual clinical expertise and patient preferences with the best available external clinical evidence from systematic research and consideration of available resources.
Evidence-Based Medicine (EBM)	EBM can be considered a subcategory of evidence-based health care, which also includes other branches of health care practice such as evidence-based nursing or evidence-based physiotherapy. EBM subcategories include evidence-based surgery and evidence-based cardiology. See also Evidence-Based Health Care.
Evidence-Based Policy Making	Policy making is evidence based when practice policies (eg, use of resources by clinicians), service policies (eg, resource allocation, pattern of services), and governance policies (eg, organizational and financial structures) are based on research evidence of benefit or cost-benefit.
Evidence-Based Practice (EBP)	EBP is clinical practice in which patient management decisions are consistent with the principles of evidence-based health care. This means that decisions will be, first of all, consistent with the best evidence about the benefits and downsides of the alternative management strategies. Second, decisions will be consistent with the values and preferences of the individual patient.

Term	Definition
Evidence-Based Practitioners	Clinicians who can differentiate evidence-based summaries and recommendations from those that are not evidence-based and understand results sufficiently well to apply them judiciously in clinical care, ensuring decisions are consistent with patients' values and preferences.
Exclusion Criteria	The characteristics that render potential participants ineligible to participate in a study or that render studies ineligible for inclusion in a systematic review.
Expectation Bias	See Bias.
Experimental Event Rate (EER)	Proportion or percentage of study participants in the experimental or intervention group in whom an event is observed.
Experimental Therapy (or Experimental Treatment or Experimental Intervention)	A therapeutic alternative to standard or control therapy, which is often a new intervention or different dose of a standard drug.
Exposure	A condition to which patients are exposed (either a potentially harmful intervention or a potentially beneficial one) that may affect their health.
External Validity (or Generalizability)	The degree to which the results of a study can be generalized to settings or samples other than the ones studied.
Face Validity	The extent to which a measurement instrument appears to measure what it is intended to measure.
Fail-Safe N	The minimum number of undetected studies with negative results that would be needed to change the conclusions of a meta-analysis. A small fail-safe N suggests that the conclusion of the meta-analysis may be susceptible to publication bias.
False Negative	Those who have the target disorder, but the test incorrectly identifies them as not having it.
False Positive	Those who do not have the target disorder, but the test incorrectly identifies them as having it.
Feedback Effect	The improvement seen in medical decision because of performance evaluation and feedback.

Term	Definition
Feeling Thermometer	A feeling thermometer is a visual analogue scale presented as a thermometer, typically with markings from 0 to 100, with 0 representing death and 100 full health. Respondents use the thermometer to indicate their utility rating of their health state or of a hypothetical health state.
Field Observation	In qualitative research, this is one of 3 basic data collection methods. It involves investigators witnessing and recording events as they occur. There are 3 approaches to field observation. With direct observation, investigators record detailed field notes from the milieu they are studying. In nonparticipant observation, the researcher participates relatively little in the interactions he or she is studying. In participant observation, the researcher assumes a role in the social setting beyond that of a researcher (eg, clinician, committee member).
Fixed-Effects Models	A model to generate a summary estimate of the magnitude of effect in a meta-analysis that restricts inferences to the set of studies included in the meta-analysis and assumes that a single true value underlies all of the primary study results. The assumption is that if all studies were infinitely large, they would yield identical estimates of effect; thus, observed estimates of effect differ from one another only because of random error. This model takes only within-study variation into account and not between-study variation.
Focus Group	See Interview.
Follow-up (or Complete Follow-up)	The extent to which investigators are aware of the outcome in every patient who participated in a study. If follow-up is complete, the outcome is known for all study participants.
Foreground Questions	These clinical questions are more commonly asked by seasoned clinicians. They are questions asked when browsing the literature (eg, what important new information should I know to optimally treat my patients?) or when problem solving (eg, defining specific questions raised in caring for patients, and then consulting the literature to resolve these problems).

Term	Definition
Funnel Plot	A graphic technique for assessing the possibility of publication bias in a systematic review. The effect measure is typically plotted on the horizontal axis and a measure of the random error associated with each study on the vertical axis. In the absence of publication bias, because of sampling variability, the graph should have the shape of a funnel. If there is bias against the publication of null results or results showing an adverse effect of the intervention, one quadrant of the funnel plot will be partially or completely missing.
Generalizability (or External Validity)	See External Validity.
Generic Health-Related Quality of Life	See Health-Related Quality of Life.
Gold Standard (or Reference Standard or Criterion Standard)	See Criterion Standard.
Grounded Theory	In qualitative research, an approach to collecting and analyzing data with the aim of developing a theory grounded in real-world observations.
Harm	Adverse consequences of exposure to an intervention.
Hawthorne Effect	The tendency for human performance to improve when participants are aware that their behavior is being observed.
Hazard Ratio	The weighted relative risk of an outcome (eg, death) during the entire study period; often reported in the context of survival analysis.
Health Costs (or Health Care Costs)	Health care resources that are consumed. These reflect the inability to use the same resources for other worthwhile purposes (opportunity costs).
Health Outcomes	All possible changes in health status that may occur for a defined population or that may be associated with exposure to an intervention. These include changes in the length and quality of life, major morbid events, and mortality.

Term	Definition
Health Profile	A type of data collection tool, intended for use in the entire population (including the healthy, the very sick, and patients with any sort of health problem), that attempts to measure all important aspects of health-related quality of life (HRQL).
Health-Related Quality of Life (HRQL)	1. Health-Related Quality of Life: Measurements of how people are feeling, or the value they place on their health state. Such measurements can be disease specific or generic. 2. Disease-Specific Health-Related Quality of Life: Disease-specific HRQL measures evaluate the full range of patients' problems and experiences relevant to a specific condition or disease. 3. Generic Health-Related Quality of Life: Generic HRQL measures contain items covering all relevant areas of HRQL. They are designed for administration to people with any kind of underlying health problem (or no problem at all). Generic HRQL measures allow comparisons across diseases or conditions.
Health State	The health condition of an individual or group during a specified interval (commonly assessed at a particular point).
Heterogeneity	Differences among individual studies included in a systematic review, typically referring to study results; the terms can also be applied to other study characteristics.
Hierarchic Regression	Hierarchic regression examines the relation between independent variables or predictor variables (eg, age, sex, disease severity) and a dependent variable (or outcome variable) (eg, death, exercise capacity). Hierarchic regression differs from standard regression in that one predictor is a subcategory of another predictor. The lower-level predictor is nested within the higher-level predictor. For instance, in a regression predicting likelihood of withdrawal of life support in intensive care units (ICUs) participating in an international study, city is nested within country and ICU is nested within city.

Term	Definition
Hierarchy of Evidence	A system of classifying and organizing types of evidence, typically for questions of treatment and prevention. Clinicians should look for the evidence from the highest position in the hierarchy.
Historiography	A qualitative research methodology concerned with understanding both historical events and approaches to the writing of historical narratives.
I^2 Statistic	The I^2 statistic is a test of heterogeneity. I^2 can be calculated from Cochrane Q (the most commonly used heterogeneity statistic) according to the formula: $I^2 = 100\% \times$ (Cochrane Q – degrees of freedom) / Cochrane Q. Any negative values of I^2 are considered equal to 0, so that the range of I^2 values is between 0% and 100%.
Incidence	Number of new cases of disease occurring during a specified period, expressed as a proportion of the number of people at risk during that time.
Inclusion Criteria	The characteristics that define the population eligible for a study or that define the studies that will be eligible for inclusion in a systematic review.
Incorporation Bias	See Bias.
Incremental Cost-Effectiveness Ratio	The price at which additional units of benefit can be obtained.
Independent Association	When a variable is associated with an outcome after adjusting for multiple other potential prognostic factors (often after regression analysis), the association is an independent association.
Independent Variable	The variable that is believed to cause, influence, or at least be associated with the dependent variable.
Indicator Condition	A clinical situation (eg, disease, symptom, injury, or health state) that occurs reasonably frequently and for which there is sound evidence that high-quality care is beneficial. Indicator conditions can be used to evaluate quality of care by comparing the care provided (as assessed through chart review or observation) to that which is recommended.

Term	Definition
Indirect Costs and Benefits	The effect of alternative patient management strategies on the productivity of the patient and others involved in the patient's care.
Individual Patient Data Meta-analysis	A meta-analysis in which individual patient data from each primary study are used to create pooled estimates. Such an approach can facilitate more accurate intention-to-treat analyses and informed subgroup analyses.
Informational Redundancy	In qualitative research, the point in the analysis at which new data fail to generate new themes and new information. This is considered an appropriate stopping point for data collection in most methods and an appropriate stopping point for analysis in some methods.
Informed Consent	A participant's expression (verbal or written) of willingness, after full disclosure of the risks, benefits, and other implications, to participate in a study.
Intention-to-Treat Principle	Analyzing participant outcomes according to the group to which they were randomized, even if participants in that group did not receive the planned intervention. This principle preserves the power of randomization, thus ensuring that important known and unknown factors that influence outcomes are likely to be equally distributed across comparison groups. We do not use the term *intention-to-treat analysis* because of ambiguity created by patients lost to follow-up, which can cause exactly the same sort of bias as failure to adhere to the intention-to-treat principle.
Internal Validity	Whether a study provides valid results depends on whether it was designed and conducted well enough that the study findings accurately represent the direction and magnitude of the underlying true effect (ie, studies that have higher internal validity have a lower likelihood of bias/systematic error).
Interrater Reliability	The extent to which 2 or more raters are able to consistently differentiate subjects with higher and lower values on an underlying trait (typically measured with an intraclass correlation).

Term	Definition
Interrupted Time Series Design (or Time Series Design)	See Time Series Design.
Interval Data (or Continuous Variable)	See Continuous Variable.
Intervention Effect (or Treatment Effect)	See Treatment Effect.
Interview	In qualitative research, this is one of 3 basic data collection methods. It involves an interviewer asking questions to engage participants in dialogue to allow interpretation of experiences and events in the participants' own terms. The 2 most common interviews are semistructured, detailed interviews of individuals or discussion-based interviews of several people, called focus groups. In quantitative research, a method of collecting data in which an interviewer obtains information from a participant through conversation.
Interviewer Bias	See Bias.
Intraclass Correlation Coefficient	This is a measure of reproducibility that compares variance between patients to the total variance, including both between- and within-patient variance.
Intrarater Reliability	The extent to which a rater is able to consistently differentiate participants with higher and lower values of an underlying trait on repeated ratings over time (typically measured with an intraclass correlation).
Inverse Rule of 3s	A rough rule of thumb, called the inverse rule of 3s, tells us the following: If an event occurs, on average, once every x days, we need to observe 3x days to be 95% confident of observing at least 1 event.
Investigator Triangulation	See Triangulation.

Term	Definition
Judgmental Sampling (or Purposive Sampling or Purposeful Sampling)	See Purposive Sampling.
Kaplan-Meier Curve (or Survival Curve)	See Survival Curve.
κ Statistic (or Weighted κ or κ Value)	A measure of the extent to which observers achieve agreement beyond the level expected to occur by chance alone.
Law of Multiplicative Probabilities	The law of multiplicative probabilities for independent events (where one event in no way influences the other) tells us that the probability of 10 consecutive heads in 10 coin flips can be found by multiplying the probability of a single head (1/2) 10 times over; that is, 1/2, 1/2, 1/2, and so on.
Leading Hypothesis (or Working Diagnosis)	See Working Diagnosis.
Lead Time Bias	See Bias.
Length Time Bias	See Bias.
Levels of Evidence	A hierarchy of research evidence to inform practice, usually ranging from strongest to weakest.
Likelihood Ratio (LR)	For a screening or diagnostic test (including clinical signs or symptoms), the LR expresses the relative likelihood that a given test would be expected in a patient with, as opposed to one without, a disorder of interest. An LR of 1 means that the posttest probability is identical to the pretest probability. As LRs increase above 1, the posttest probability progressively increases in relation to the pretest probability. As LRs decrease below 1, the posttest probability progressively decreases in relation to the pretest probability. An LR is calculated as the proportion of target positive with a particular test result (which, with a single cut point, would be either a positive or negative result) divided by the proportion of target negative with same test result.

Term	Definition
Likert Scales	Scales, typically with 3 to 9 possible values, that include extremes of attitudes or feelings (such as from totally disagree to totally agree) that respondents mark to indicate their rating.
Linear Regression	The term used for a regression analysis when the dependent variable or target variable is a continuous variable and the relationship between the dependent variable and independent variable is thought to be linear.
Local Consensus Process	A strategy for changing clinician behavior. Inclusion of participating clinicians in discussions to create agreement with a suggested approach to change provider practice.
Local Opinion Leaders (or Opinion Leaders)	A strategy for changing clinician behavior. These persons are clinician peers who are recognized by their colleagues as model caregivers or who are viewed as having particular content expertise.
Logical Operators (or Boolean Operators)	See Boolean Operators.
Logistic Regression	A regression analysis in which the dependent variable is binary.
Longitudinal Study (or Cohort Study or Prospective Study)	See Cohort Study.
Lost to Follow-up	Patients whose status on the outcome or endpoint of interest is unknown.
Markov Model (or Multistate Transition Model)	Markov models are tools used in decision analyses. Named after a 19th-century Russian mathematician, Markov models are the basis of software programs that model what might happen to a cohort of patients during a series of cycles (eg, periods of 1 year). The model allows for the possibility that patients might move from one health state to another. For instance, one patient may have a mild stroke in one 3-month cycle, continue with minimal functional limitation for a number of cycles, have a gastrointestinal bleeding episode in a subsequent cycle, and finally experience a major stroke. Ideally, data from randomized trials will determine the probability of moving from one state to another during any cycle under competing management options.

Term	Definition
Masked (or Blind or Blinded)	See Blind.
Matching	A deliberate process to make the intervention group and comparison group comparable with respect to factors (or confounders) that are extraneous to the purpose of the investigation but that might interfere with the interpretation of the study's findings. For example, in case-control studies, individual cases may be matched with controls on the basis of comparable age, sex, or other clinical features.
Median Survival	Length of time that half the study population survives.
Medical Subject Headings (MeSH)	The National Library of Medicine's controlled vocabulary used for indexing articles for MEDLINE/ PubMed. MeSH terminology provides a consistent way to retrieve information that may use different terminologies for the same concepts.
Member Checking	In qualitative research, this involves sharing draft study findings with the participants to inquire whether their viewpoints were faithfully interpreted and to ascertain whether the account makes sense to participants.
Meta-analysis	A statistical technique for quantitatively combining the results of multiple studies measuring the same outcome into a single pooled or summary estimate.
Meta-Regression Analysis	When summarizing patient or design characteristics at the individual trial level, meta-analysts risk failing to detect genuine relationships between these characteristics and the size of treatment effect. Further, the risk of obtaining a spurious explanation for variable treatment effects is high when the number of trials is small and many patient and design characteristics differ. Meta-regression techniques can be used to explore whether patient characteristics (eg, younger or older patients) or design characteristics (eg, studies of low or high quality) are related to the size of the treatment effect.

Term	Definition
Meta-Synthesis	A procedure for combining qualitative research on a specific topic in which researchers compare and analyze the texts of individual studies and develop new interpretations.
Minimal Important Difference	The smallest difference in a patient-important outcome that patients perceive as beneficial and that would mandate, in the absence of troublesome adverse effects and excessive cost, a change in the patient's health care management.
Mixed-Methods Study	A study that combines data collection approaches, sometimes both qualitative and quantitative, into the study methodology and is commonly used in the study of service delivery and organization. Some mixed-methods studies combine study designs (eg, investigators may embed qualitative or quantitative process evaluations alongside quantitative evaluative designs to increase understanding of factors influencing a phenomenon) Some mixed-methods studies include a single overarching research design but use mixed-methods for data collection (eg, surveys, interviews, observation, and analysis of documentary material).
Model	The term *model* is often used to describe statistical regression analyses involving more than 1 independent variable and 1 dependent variable. This is a multivariable or multiple regression (or multivariate) analysis.
Multifaceted Interventions	Use of multiple strategies to change clinician behavior. Multiple strategies may include a combination that includes 2 or more of the following: audit and feedback, reminders, local consensus processes, patient-mediated interventions, or computer decision support systems.
Multistate Transition Model	See Markov Model.
Multivariate Regression Analysis (or Multivariable Analysis or Multivariable Regression Equation)	A type of regression that provides a mathematical model that attempts to explain or predict the dependent variable (or outcome variable or target variable) by simultaneously considering 2 or more independent variables (or predictor variables).

Term	Definition
n-of-1 Randomized Controlled Trial (or n-of-1 RCT)	An experiment designed to determine the effect of an intervention or exposure on a single study participant. In one n-of-1 design, the patient undergoes pairs of treatment periods organized so that 1 period involves the use of the experimental treatment and 1 period involves the use of an alternate treatment or placebo. The patient and clinician are blinded if possible, and outcomes are monitored. Treatment periods are replicated until the clinician and patient are convinced that the treatments are definitely different or definitely not different.
Narrative Review	A review article (such as a typical book chapter) that is not conducted using methods to minimize bias (in contrast to a systematic review).
Natural History	As distinct from prognosis, natural history refers to the possible consequences and outcomes of a disease or condition and the frequency with which they can be expected to occur when the disease condition is untreated.
Negative Predictive Value (NPV)	See Predictive Value.
Negative Study (or Negative Trial)	Studies in which the authors have concluded that the comparison groups do not differ statistically in the variables of interest. Research results that fail to support the researchers' hypotheses.
Neural Network	The application of nonlinear statistics to pattern-recognition problems. Neural networks can be used to develop clinical prediction rules. The technique identifies those predictors most strongly associated with the outcome of interest that belong in a clinical prediction rule and those that can be omitted from the rule without loss of predictive power.
Nomogram	Graphic scale facilitating calculation of a probability. The most-used nomogram in the EBM world is one developed by Fagan to move from a pretest probability, through a likelihood ratio, to a posttest probability.
Nonadherent	Patients are nonadherent if they are not exposed to the full course of a study intervention (eg, most commonly, they do not take the prescribed dose or duration of a drug or they do not participate fully in the study program).

Term	Definition
Noninferiority Trial (or Equivalence Trial)	Trials that estimate treatment effects that exclude any patient-important superiority of the control intervention under evaluation are noninferiority trials. Noninferiority trials require a previous definition of the smallest difference in outcomes between the interventions that patients would consider large enough in favor of the control group to justify a preference for the control intervention. The confidence interval for the estimated treatment effect at the end of the trial should exclude that difference in favor of the control group for the authors to claim noninferiority (ie, the upper limit of the confidence interval should be closer to zero than the minimal patient important difference). This level of precision requires fewer patients and events than an equivalence trial. Noninferiority trials are helpful when investigators want to see whether a cheaper, safer, simpler intervention is better than or the same (is not worse in terms of efficacy) as what is done currently
Nonparticipant Observation	See Field Observation.
Null Hypothesis	In the hypothesis-testing framework, this is the starting hypothesis that the statistical test is designed to consider and possibly reject, which contends that there is no relationship between the variables under study.
Null Result	A nonsignificant result; no statistically significant difference between groups.
Number Needed to Harm (NNH)	The number of patients who, if they received the experimental intervention, would lead to 1 additional patient being harmed during a specific period. It is the inverse of the absolute risk increase (ARI), expressed as a percentage (100/ARI).
Number Needed to Screen (NNS)	The number of patients who would need to be screened to prevent 1 adverse event.
Number Needed to Treat (NNT)	The number of patients who need to be treated during a specific period to achieve 1 additional good outcome. When NNT is discussed, it is important to specify the intervention, its duration, and the desirable outcome. It is the inverse of the absolute risk reduction (ARR), expressed as a percentage (100/ARR).

Term	Definition
Observational Study (or Observational Study Design)	An observational study can be used to describe many designs that are not randomized trials (eg, cohort studies or case-control studies that have a goal of establishing causation, studies of prognosis, studies of diagnostic tests, and qualitative studies). The term is most often used in the context of cohort studies and case-control studies in which patient or caregiver preference, or happenstance, determines whether a person is exposed to an intervention or putative harmful agent or behavior (in contrast to the exposure's being under the control of the investigator, as in a randomized trial).
Observer Bias	See Bias.
Odds	The ratio of events to nonevents; the ratio of the number of study participants experiencing the outcome of interest to the number of study participants not experiencing the outcome of interest.
Odds Ratio (OR) (or Relative Odds)	A ratio of the odds of an event in an exposed group to the odds of the same event in a group that is not exposed.
Odds Reduction	The odds reduction expresses, for odds, what relative risk reduction expresses for risks. Just as the relative risk reduction is 1 − relative risk, the odds reduction is 1 − relative odds (the relative odds and odds ratio being synonymous). Thus, if a treatment results in an odds ratio of 0.6 for a particular outcome, the treatment reduces the odds for that outcome by 0.4.
One-Group Pre-test-Posttest Design (or Before-After Design)	See Before-After Design.
Open-Ended Questions	Questions that offer no specific structure for the respondents' answers and allow the respondents to answer in their own words.
Opinion Leaders (or Local Opinion Leaders)	See Local Opinion Leaders.

Term	Definition
Opportunity Costs	The value of (health or other) benefits forgone in alternative uses when a resource is used.
Outcome Variable (or Dependent Variable or Target Variable)	The target variable of interest. The variable that is hypothesized to depend on or be caused by another variable (the independent variable).
Partial Verification Bias	See Bias.
Participant Observation	See Field Observation.
Patient-Important Outcomes	Outcomes that patients value directly. This is in contrast to surrogate, substitute, or physiologic outcomes that clinicians may consider important. One way of thinking about a patient-important outcome is that, were it to be the only thing that changed, patients would be willing to undergo a treatment with associated risk, cost, or inconvenience. This would be true of treatments that ameliorated symptoms or prevented morbidity or mortality. It would not be true of treatments that lowered blood pressure, improved cardiac output, improved bone density, or the like, without improving the quality or increasing the length of life.
Patient-Mediated Interventions	A strategy for changing clinician behavior. Any intervention aimed at changing the performance of health care professionals through interactions with, or information provided by or to, patients.
Patient Preferences	The relative value that patients place on various health states. Preferences are determined by values, beliefs, and attitudes that patients bring to bear in considering what they will gain—or lose—as a result of a management decision. Explicit enumeration and balancing of benefits and risks that is central to evidence-based clinical practice brings the underlying value judgments involved in making management decisions into bold relief.

Term	Definition
Per-Protocol Analysis	An analysis restricted to patients who adhered to their assigned treatment in a randomized trial (omitting patients who dropped out of the study or for other reasons did not actually receive the planned intervention). This analysis can provide a misleading estimate of effect because all patients randomized are no longer included, raising concerns about whether important unknown factors that influence outcome are equally distributed across comparison groups.
Phase I Studies	Studies often conducted in normal volunteers that investigate a drug's physiologic effect and evaluate whether it manifests unacceptable early toxicity.
Phase II Studies	Initial studies on patients that provide preliminary evidence of possible drug effectiveness.
Phase III Studies	Randomized controlled trials designed to test the magnitude of benefit and harm of a drug.
Phase IV Studies (or Postmarketing Surveillance Studies)	Studies conducted after the effectiveness of a drug has been established and the drug marketed, typically to establish the frequency of uncommon or unanticipated toxic effects.
Phenomenology	In qualitative research, an approach to inquiry that emphasizes the complexity of human experience and the need to understand the experience holistically as it is actually lived.
φ (Or φ Statistic)	A measure of chance-independent agreement.
PICO (or Patient, Intervention, Comparison, Outcome)	A method for answering clinical questions.
Placebo	A biologically inert substance (typically a pill or capsule) that is as similar as possible to the active intervention. Placebos are sometimes given to participants in the control arm of a drug trial to help ensure that the study is blinded.
Placebo Effect	The effect of an intervention independent of its biologic effect.

Term	Definition
Point Estimate	The single value that best represents the value of the population parameter.
Pooled Estimate	A statistical summary measure representing the best estimate of a parameter that applies to all the studies that contribute to addressing a similar question (such as a pooled relative risk and 95% confidence intervals from a set of randomized trials).
Positive Predictive Value (PPV)	See Predictive Value.
Positive Study (or Positive Trial)	A study with results that show a difference that investigators interpret as beyond the play of chance.
Posttest Odds	The odds of the target condition being present after the results of a diagnostic test are available.
Posttest Probability	The probability of the target condition being present after the results of a diagnostic test are available.
Power	The ability of a study to reject a null hypothesis when it is false (and should be rejected). Power is linked to the adequacy of the sample size: if a sample size is too small, the study will have insufficient power to detect differences between groups.
Practice Guidelines (or Clinical Practice Guidelines or Guidelines)	See Clinical Practice Guidelines.
Prediction Rules (or Clinical Prediction Rules)	See Clinical Prediction Rules.
Predictive Value	Two categories: Positive predictive value—the proportion of people with a positive test result who have the disease; negative predictive value—the proportion of people with a negative test result and who are free of disease.
Preferences	See Values and Preferences.

Term	Definition
Pretest Odds	The odds of the target condition being present before the results of a diagnostic test are available.
Pretest Probability	The probability of the target condition being present before the results of a diagnostic test are available.
Prevalence	Proportion of persons affected with a particular disease at a specified time. Prevalence rates obtained from high-quality studies can inform pretest probabilities.
Prevent (Prevention)	A preventive maneuver is an action that decreases the risk of a future event or the threatened onset of disease. Primary prevention is designed to stop a condition from developing. Secondary prevention is designed to stop or slow progression of a disease or disorder when patients have a disease and are at risk for developing something related to their current disease. Often, secondary prevention is indistinguishable from treatment. An example of primary prevention is vaccination for pertussis. An example of secondary prevention is administration of an antiosteoporosis intervention to women with low bone density and evidence of a vertebral fracture to prevent subsequent fractures. An example of tertiary prevention is a rehabilitation program for patients experiencing the adverse effects associated with a myocardial infarction.
Primary Studies	Studies that collect original data. Primary studies are differentiated from synopses that summarize the results of individual primary studies and they are different from systematic reviews that summarize the results of a number of primary studies.
Probability	Quantitative estimate of the likelihood of a condition existing (as in diagnosis) or of subsequent events (such as in an intervention study).
Prognosis	The possible consequences and outcomes of a disease and the frequency with which they can be expected to occur.
Prognostic Factors	Patient or participant characteristics that confer increased or decreased risk of a positive or adverse outcome.

Term	Definition
Prognostic Study	A study that enrolls patients at a point in time and follows them forward to determine the frequency and timing of subsequent events.
Prospective Study (or Cohort Study or Longitudinal Study)	See Cohort Study.
Publication Bias	See Bias.
Purposive Sampling (or Purposeful Sampling or Judgmental Sampling)	In qualitative research, a type of nonprobability sampling in which theory or personal judgment guides the selection of study participants. Depending on the topic, examples include maximum variation sampling to document range or diversity; extreme case sampling, in which one selects cases that are opposite in some way; typical or representative case sampling to describe what is common in terms of the phenomenon of interest; critical sampling to make a point dramatically; and criterion sampling, in which all cases that meet some predetermined criteria of importance are studied.
P Value (or P)	The probability that results as extreme as or more extreme than those observed would occur if the null hypothesis were true and the experiment were repeated over and over. $P < .05$ means that there is a less than 1 in 20 probability that, on repeated performance of the experiment, the results as extreme as or more extreme than those observed would occur if the null hypothesis were true.
Qualitative Research	Qualitative research focuses on social and interpreted, rather than quantifiable, phenomena and aims to discover, interpret, and describe rather than to test and evaluate. Qualitative research makes inductive, descriptive inferences to theory concerning social experiences or settings, whereas quantitative research makes causal or correlational inferences to populations. Qualitative research is not a single method but a family of analytic approaches that rely on the description and interpretation of qualitative data. Specific methods include, for example, grounded theory, ethnography, phenomenology, case study, critical theory, and historiography.

Term	Definition
Quality-Adjusted Life-Year (QALY)	A unit of measure for survival that accounts for the effects of suboptimal health status and the resulting limitations in quality of life. For example, if a patient lives for 10 years and his or her quality of life is decreased by 50% because of chronic lung disease, survival would be equivalent to 5 QALYs.
Quality Improvement	An approach to defining, measuring, improving, and controlling practices to maintain or improve the appropriateness of health care services.
Quality of Care	The extent to which health care meets technical and humanistic standards of optimal care.
Quantitative Research	The investigation of phenomena that lend themselves to test well-specified hypotheses through precise measurement and quantification of predetermined variables that yield numbers suitable for statistical analysis.
Random	Governed by a formal chance process in which the occurrence of previous events is of no value in predicting future events. For example, the probability of assigning a participant to one of 2 specified groups is 50%.
Random Allocation (or Randomization)	See Randomization.
Random-Effects Model	A model used to give a summary estimate of the magnitude of effect in a meta-analysis that assumes that the studies included are a random sample of a population of studies addressing the question posed in the meta-analysis. Each study estimates a different underlying true effect, and the distribution of these effects is assumed to be normal around a mean value. Because a random-effects model takes into account both within-study and between-study variability, the confidence interval around the point estimate is, when there is appreciable variability in results across studies, wider than it could be if a fixed-effects model were used.

Term	Definition
Random Error (or Chance)	We can never know with certainty the true value of an intervention effect because of random error. It is inherent in all measurement. The observations that are made in a study are only a sample of all possible observations that could be made from the population of relevant patients. Thus, the average value of any sample of observations is subject to some variation from the true value for that entire population. When the level of random error associated with a measurement is high, the measurement is less precise and we are less certain about the value of that measurement.
Randomization (or Random Allocation)	Allocation of participants to groups by chance, usually done with the aid of a table of random numbers. Not to be confused with systematic allocation or quasi-randomization (eg, on even and odd days of the month) or other allocation methods at the discretion of the investigator.
Randomized Controlled Trial (RCT) (or Randomized Trial)	Experiment in which individuals are randomly allocated to receive or not receive an experimental diagnostic, preventive, therapeutic, or palliative procedure and then followed to determine the effect of the intervention.
Randomized Trial (or Randomized Controlled Trial)	See Randomized Controlled Trial.
Random Sample	A sample derived by selecting sampling units (eg, individual patients) such that each unit has an independent and fixed (generally equal) chance of selection. Whether a given unit is selected is determined by chance; for example, by a table of randomly ordered numbers.
Recall Bias	See Bias.
Receiver Operating Characteristic Curve (or ROC Curve)	A figure depicting the power of a diagnostic test. The ROC curve presents the test's true-positive rate (ie, sensitivity) on the horizontal axis and the false-positive rate (ie, 1 − specificity) on the vertical axis for different cut points dividing a positive from a negative test. An ROC curve for a perfect test has an area under the curve of 1.0, whereas a test that performs no better than chance has an area under the curve of only 0.5.

Term	Definition
Recursive Partitioning Analysis	A technique for determining the optimal way of using a set of predictor variables to estimate the likelihood of an individual's experiencing a particular outcome. The technique repeatedly divides the population (eg, old vs young; among young and old) according to status on variables that discriminate between those who will have the outcome of interest and those who will not.
Reference Standard (or Gold Standard or Criterion Standard)	See Criterion Standard.
Referral Bias	See Bias.
Reflexivity	In qualitative research using field observation, whichever of the 3 approaches used, the observer will always have some effect on what is being observed, small or large. This interaction of the observer with what is observed is called reflexivity. Whether it plays a positive or negative role in accessing social truths, the researcher must acknowledge and investigate reflexivity and account for it in data interpretation.
Regression (or Regression Analysis)	A technique that uses predictor or independent variables to build a statistical model that predicts an individual patient's status with respect to a dependent variable or target variable.
Relative Diagnostic Odds Ratio	The diagnostic odds ratio is a single value that provides one way of representing the power of the diagnostic test. It is applicable when we have a single cut point for a test and classify tests results as positive and negative. The diagnostic odds ratio is calculated as the product of the true positive and true negative divided by the product of the false positives and false negatives. The relative diagnostic odds ratio is the ratio of one diagnostic odds ratio to another.
Relative Odds	See Odds Ratio. Just as relative risk and risk ratio are synonymous, relative odds and odds ratio are synonymous.
Relative Risk (RR) (or Risk Ratio)	Ratio of the risk of an event among an exposed population to the risk among the unexposed.

Term	Definition
Relative Risk Increase (RRI)	The proportional increase in rates of harmful outcomes between experimental and control participants. It is calculated by dividing the rate of harmful outcome in the experimental group (experimental event rate, or EER) minus the rate of harmful outcome in the control group (control event rate, or CER) by the rate of harmful outcome in the control group ([EER – CER]/CER). Typically used with a harmful exposure.
Relative Risk Reduction (RRR)	The proportional reduction in rates of harmful outcomes between experimental and control participants. It is calculated by dividing the rate of harmful outcome in the control group (control event rate, or CER) minus the rate of harmful outcome in the experimental group (experimental event rate, or EER) by the rate of harmful outcome in the control group ([CER – EER]/ CER). Used with a beneficial exposure or intervention.
Reliability	Reliability is used as a technical statistical term that refers to a measurement instrument's ability to differentiate between subjects, patients, or participants in some underlying trait. Reliability increases as the variability between subjects increases and decreases as the variability within subjects (over time, or over raters) increases. Reliability is typically expressed as an intraclass correlation coefficient with between-subject variability in the numerator and total variability (between-subject and within-subject) in the denominator.
Reminding (or Reminders or Reminder Systems)	A strategy for changing clinician behavior. Manual or computerized reminders to prompt behavior change.
Reporting Bias (or Selective Outcome Reporting Bias)	See Bias.
Residual Confounding	Unknown, unmeasured, or suboptimally measured prognostic factors that remain unbalanced between groups after full covariable adjustment by statistical techniques. The remaining imbalance will lead to a biased assessment of the effect of any putatively causal exposure.

Term	Definition
Responsiveness	The sensitivity or ability of an instrument to detect change over time.
Review	A general term for articles that summarize the results of more than 1 primary study. See also Systematic Review.
Risk	A measure of the association between exposure and outcome (including incidence, adverse effects, or toxicity).
Risk Factors	Risk factors are patient characteristics associated with the development of a disease in the first place. Prognostic factors are patient characteristics that confer increased or decreased risk of a positive or adverse outcome from a given disease.
Risk Ratio (or Relative Risk)	See Relative Risk.
Screening	Services designed to detect people at high risk of experiencing a condition associated with a modifiable adverse outcome, offered to persons who have neither symptoms of nor risk factors for a target condition.
Secondary Journal	A secondary journal does not publish original research but rather includes synopses of published research studies that meet prespecified criteria of both clinical relevance and methodologic quality.
Secular Trends	Changes in the probability of events with time, independent of known predictors of outcome.
Semistructured Interview	In qualitative research, the interviewer asks a number of specific questions, but additional questions or probes are used at the discretion of the interviewer.
Sensitivity	The proportion of people who truly have a designated disorder who are so identified by the test. The test may consist of, or include, clinical observations.
Sensitivity Analysis	Any test of the stability of the conclusions of a health care evaluation over a range of probability estimates, value judgments, and assumptions about the structure of the decisions to be made. This may involve the repeated evaluation of a decision model in which one or more of the parameters of interest are varied.

Term	Definition
Sentinel Effect	The tendency for human performance to improve when participants are aware that their behavior is being evaluated; in contrast to the Hawthorne effect, which refers to behavior change as a result of being observed but not evaluated.
Sequential Sample (or Consecutive Sample)	See Consecutive Sample.
Sign	Any abnormality indicative of disease, discoverable by the clinician at an examination of the patient. It is an objective aspect of a disease.
Signal-to-Noise Ratio	Signal refers to the target of the measurement; noise, to random error that obscures the signal. When one is trying to discriminate among people at a single point in time (who is better off, who is worse off) the signal comes from differences in scores between patients. The noise comes from variability or differences in score within patients over time. The greater the noise, the more difficult it is to detect the signal. When one is trying to evaluate change over time, the signal comes from the difference in scores in patients whose status has improved or deteriorated. The noise comes from the variability in scores in patients whose status has not changed.
Sign Test	A nonparametric test for comparing 2 paired groups according to the relative ranking of values between the pairs.
Silo Effect	One of the main reasons for considering narrower viewpoints in conducting an economic analysis is to assess the effect of change on the main budget holders because budgets may need to be adjusted before a new intervention can be adopted (the silo effect).
Simple Regression (or Univariate Regression)	See Univariable Regression.
Social Desirability Bias	See Bias.

Term	Definition
Specificity	The proportion of people who are truly free of a designated disorder who are so identified by the test. The test may consist of, or include, clinical observations.
Spectrum Bias	See Bias.
Stakeholder Analysis	A strategy that seeks to increase understanding of stakeholder behavior, plans, relationships, and interests and seeks to generate information about stakeholders' levels of influence, support, and resources.
Standard Error	The standard deviation of an estimate of a population parameter. The standard error of the mean is the standard deviation of the estimate of the population mean value.
Standard Gamble	A direct preference or utility measure that effectively asks respondents to rate their quality of life on a scale from 0 to 1.0, where 0 is death and 1.0 is full health. Respondents choose between a specified time x in their current health state and a gamble in which they have probability P (anywhere from 0 to .99) of full health for time x, and a probability $1 - P$ of immediate death.
Statistical Significance	A term indicating that the results obtained in an analysis of study data are unlikely to have occurred by chance and the null hypothesis is rejected. When statistically significant, the probability of the observed results, given the null hypothesis, falls below a specified level of probability (most often $P < .05$).
Stopped Early Trials (Truncated Trials)	Truncated randomized controlled trials (RCTs) are trials stopped early because of apparent harm because the investigators have concluded that they will not be able to demonstrate a treatment effect (futility), or because of apparent benefit. Believing the treatment from RCTs stopped early for benefit will be misleading if the decision to stop the trial resulted from catching the apparent benefit of treatment at a random high.

Term	Definition
Stopping Rules	These are methodologic and statistical guides that inform decisions to stop trials early. They can incorporate issues such as the planned sample size, planned and conducted interim analyses, presence and type of data monitoring including independent research oversight, statistical boundaries, and statistical adjustments for interim analyses and stopping.
Structured Abstract	A brief summary of the key elements of an article following pre-specified headings. For example, the *ACP Journal Club* therapy abstracts include major headings of question, methods, setting, patients, intervention, main results, and conclusion. More highly structured abstracts include sub-headings. For example, *ACP Journal Club* therapy abstracts methods sections include design, allocation, blinding, and follow-up period.
Subgroup Analysis	The separate analysis of data for subgroups of patients, such as those at different stages of their illness, those with different comorbid conditions, or those of different ages.
Substitute Outcomes or Endpoints (or Surrogate Outcomes or Endpoints)	See Surrogate Endpoints.
Surrogate Outcomes or Endpoints (or Substitute Outcomes or Endpoints)	Outcomes that are not in themselves important to patients but are associated with outcomes that are important to patients (eg, bone density for fracture, cholesterol for myocardial infarction, and blood pressure for stroke). These outcomes would not influence patient behavior if they were the only outcomes that would change with an intervention.
Surveillance Bias	See Bias.
Survey	Observational study that focuses on obtaining information about activities, beliefs, preferences, knowledge, or attitudes from respondents through interviewer-administered or self-administered methods.

Term	Definition
Survival Analysis	A statistical procedure used to compare the proportion of patients in each group who experience an outcome or endpoint at various intervals throughout the duration of the study (eg, death).
Survival Curve (or Kaplan-Meier Curve)	A curve that starts at 100% of the study population and shows the percentage of the population still surviving (or free of disease or some other outcome) at successive times for as long as information is available.
Symptom	Any phenomenon or departure from the normal in function, appearance, or sensation reported by the patient and suggestive or indicative of disease.
Syndrome	A collection of signs or symptoms or physiologic abnormalities.
Synopsis	Brief summary that encapsulates the key methodologic details and results of a single study or systematic review.
Systematic Error (or Bias)	See Bias.
Systematic Review	The identification, selection, appraisal, and summary of primary studies addressing a focused clinical question using methods to reduce the likelihood of bias.
Systems	Systems include practice guidelines, clinical pathways, or evidence-based textbook summaries that integrate evidence-based information about specific clinical problems and provide regular updates to guide the care of individual patients.
Target Condition	In diagnostic test studies, the condition the investigators or clinicians are particularly interested in identifying (such as tuberculosis, lung cancer, or iron-deficiency anemia).
Target-Negative	In diagnostic test studies, patients who do not have the target condition.
Target Outcome (or Target Endpoints or Target Events)	In intervention studies, the condition the investigators or clinicians are particularly interested in identifying and in which it is anticipated the intervention will decrease (such as myocardial infarction, stroke, or death) or increase (such as ulcer healing).

Term	Definition
Target-Positive	In diagnostic test studies, patients who have the target condition.
Target Variable (or Dependent Variable or Outcome Variable)	See Dependent Variable.
Test Threshold (or No-Test Test Threshold)	The probability below which the clinician decides a diagnosis warrants no further consideration.
Theoretical Saturation	In qualitative research, this is the point in the analysis at which themes are well organized into a coherent theory or conceptual framework. This is considered an appropriate stopping point for data analysis, especially in grounded theory methods.
Theory	Theory consists of concepts and their relationships.
Theory Triangulation	See Triangulation.
Threshold NNT (or Threshold NNH)	Maximum number needed to treat (NNT) or number needed to harm (NNH) accepted as justifying the benefits and harms of therapy.
Time Series Design (or Interrupted Time Series Design)	In this study design, data are collected at several points both before and after the intervention. Data collected before the intervention allow the underlying trend and cyclical (seasonal) effects to be estimated. Data collected after the intervention allow the intervention effect to be estimated while accounting for underlying secular trends. The time series design monitors the occurrence of outcomes or end points during a number of cycles and determines whether the pattern changes coincident with the intervention.

Term	Definition
Treatment Effect (or Intervention Effect)	The results of comparative clinical studies can be expressed using various intervention effect measures. Examples are absolute risk reduction (ARR), relative risk reduction (RRR), odds ratio (OR), number needed to treat (NNT), and effect size. The appropriateness of using these to express an intervention effect and whether probabilities, means, or medians are used to calculate them depend on the type of outcome variable used to measure health outcomes. For example, ARR, RRR, and NNT are used for dichotomous variables, and effect sizes are normally used for continuous variables.
Treatment Target	The manifestation of illness (a symptom, sign, or physiologic abnormality) toward which a treatment is directed.
Treatment Threshold (or Therapeutic Threshold)	Probability above which a clinician would consider a diagnosis confirmed and would stop testing and initiate treatment.
Trial of Therapy	In a trial of therapy, the physician offers the patient an intervention, reviews the effect of the intervention on that patient at some subsequent time, and, depending on the effect, recommends either continuation or discontinuation of the intervention.
Triangulation	In qualitative research, an analytic approach in which key findings are corroborated using multiple sources of information. There are different types of triangulation. Investigator triangulation requires more than 1 investigator to collect and analyze the raw data, such that the findings emerge through consensus among a team of investigators. Theory triangulation is a process whereby emergent findings are corroborated with existing social science theories.

Term	Definition
Trim-and-Fill Method	When publication bias is suspected in a systematic review, investigators may attempt to estimate the true intervention effect by removing, or trimming, small positive-result studies that do not have a negative-result study counterpart and then calculating a supposed true effect from the resulting symmetric funnel plot. The investigators then replace the positive-result studies they have removed and add hypothetical studies that mirror these positive-result studies to create a symmetric funnel plot that retains the new pooled effect estimate. This method allows the calculation of an adjusted confidence interval and an estimate of the number of missing trials.
True Negative	Those whom the test correctly identifies as not having the target disorder.
True Positive	Those whom the test correctly identifies as having the target disorder.
Truncated Trials (Stopped Early Trials)	See Stopped Early Trials.
Trustworthiness (or Credibility)	See Credibility.
t Test	A parametric statistical test that examines the difference between the means of 2 groups of values.
Type I Error	An error created by rejecting the null hypothesis when it is true (ie, investigators conclude that a relationship exists between variables when it does not).
Type II Error	An error created by accepting the null hypothesis when it is false (ie, investigators conclude that no relationship exists between variables when, in fact, a relationship does exist).
Unblinded (or Unmasked)	Patients, clinicians, those monitoring outcomes, judicial assessors of outcomes, data analysts, and manuscript authors are aware of whether patients have been assigned to the experimental or control group.

Term	Definition
Unit of Allocation	The unit or focus used for assignment to comparison groups (eg, individuals or clusters such as schools, health care teams, hospital wards, outpatient practices).
Unit of Analysis	The unit or focus of the analysis; although it is most often the individual study participant, in a study that uses cluster allocation, the unit of analysis is the cluster (eg, school, clinic).
Unit of Analysis Error	When investigators use any sort of cluster randomization (randomize by physician instead of patient, practice instead of physician or patient, or village instead of participant) and analyze as if they have randomized according to patient or participant, they have made a unit of analysis error. The appropriate analysis acknowledges the cluster randomization and takes into account the extent to which outcomes differ between clusters independent of treatment effect.
Univariate Regression (or Univariable Regression or Simple Regression)	Regression when there is only 1 independent variable under evaluation with respect to a dependent variable.
Unmasked (or Unblinded)	See Unblinded.
Up-Front Costs	Costs incurred to "produce" the treatment such as the physician's time, nurse's time, and materials.
Utilitarian (or Consequentialist)	See Consequentialist.
Utilization Review	An organized procedure to review admissions; duration of stay; and professional, pharmacologic, or programmatic services provided and to evaluate the need for those services and promote their most efficient use.
Validity (or Credibility)	In health status measurement terms, validity is the extent to which an instrument measures what it is intended to measure. In critical appraisal terms, validity reflects the extent to which the study results are likely to be subject to systematic error and thus be more or less likely to reflect the truth. See also Credibility.

Term	Definition
Values and Preferences	When used generically, as in "values and preferences," we refer to the collection of goals, expectations, predispositions, and beliefs that individuals have for certain decisions and their potential outcomes. The incorporation of patient values and preferences in decision making is central to evidence-based medicine. These terms also carry specific meaning in other settings. Measurement tools that require a choice under conditions of uncertainty to indirectly measure preference for an outcome in health economics (such as the standard gamble) quantify preferences. Measurement tools that evaluate the outcome on a scale with defined favorable and unfavorable ends (eg, visual analog scales, feeling thermometers) quantify values.
Variance	The technical term for the statistical estimate of the variability in results.
Verification Bias	See Differential Verification Bias.
Visual Analogue Scale	A scaling procedure consisting of a straight line anchored on each end with words or phrases that represent the extremes of some phenomenon (eg, "worst pain I have ever had" to "absolutely no pain"). Respondents are asked to make a mark on the line at the point that corresponds to their experience of the phenomenon.
Washout Period	In a crossover or n-of-1 trial, the period required for the treatment to cease to act once it has been discontinued.
Working Diagnosis (or Leading Hypothesis)	The clinician's single best explanation for the patient's clinical problem(s).
Workup Bias	See Differential Verification Bias.

Index

C

S